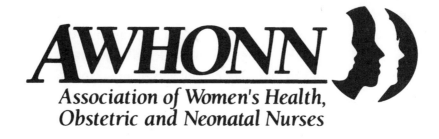

AWHONN
Association of Women's Health,
Obstetric and Neonatal Nurses

FETAL HEART MONITORING
PRINCIPLES AND PRACTICES
Second Edition

Editors

Nancy Feinstein, RNC, MSN
Patricia McCartney, RNC, PhD

Contributors

Nancy Feinstein, RNC, MSN
Susan Gilson, RNC
Tracey Kasnic, RNC, BSN
Patricia McCartney, RNC, PhD, Revisions Task Force Chair
Keiko Torgersen, RNC, BSN, MS
Catherine Weiser, RN, MS, FNP

KENDALL/HUNT PUBLISHING COMPANY
4050 Westmark Drive   Dubuque, Iowa 52002

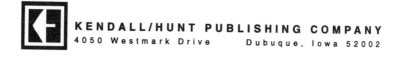

Any procedure or practice described in this book should be applied by the health care practitioner under appropriate supervision in accordance with professional standards of care used with regard to the specific circumstances of each practice situation. Care has been taken to confirm the accuracy of information presented and to describe generally accepted practices. However, the authors, editors, and publisher cannot accept any responsibility for errors or omissions or for any consequences resulting from the application of the information in this book and make no warranty, express or implied, with respect to the contents of the book.

The authors and publisher have exerted every effort to ensure that drug selection and dosage set forth in this text are in accordance with current recommendations and practice at the time of publication. However, in view of ongoing changes in government regulations, and the constant flow of information relating to drug therapy and drug reactions, the reader is urged to check the package insert for each drug for any changes in indications and dosage and for added warnings and precautions. This is particularly important when the recommended agent is a new or infrequently used drug.

AWHONN recognizes that Electronic Fetal Heart Rate Monitoring: Research Guidelines developed by the National Institute of Child Health and Human Development (NICHD) Research Planning workshop was published in 1997.* This document contains a proposed nomenclature system for electronic fetal monitoring interpretation. "Once the nomenclature is tested, refined, and determined valid, it would seem reasonable for clinicians to use the definitions in clinical practice, although it's far too early to speculate as to how these changes will affect practice."** As future trends in bedside practice evolve based on these guidelines, AWHONN will update its programs accordingly.

*The NICHD report was published concurrently in the November/December 1997 issues of AWHONN's *Journal of Obstetric, Gynecologic and Neonatal Nurses (JOGNN)* and in the *American Journal of Obstetrics and Gynecology*.

**Harvey, Carol J. (1997). Electronic fetal monitoring update: A Look at the New Terms, *Lifelines*, December 1997.

Harvey, Carol J. (1997). "Electronic fetal monitoring update: Coming to Terms," *Lifelines*, June 1997.

ACKNOWLEDGMENTS

First Edition Authors of *Fetal Heart Monitoring Principles and Practices*:

Donna Adelsperger, RNC, MEd
Julie Carr, RN, MSN
Deborah Davis, RNC, BSN
Nancy Feinstein, RNC, MSN
Judy Schmidt, RNC, EdD, Chair

Our most sincere appreciation goes to the original authors, who also served on the Fetal Heart Monitoring Education Program Steering Committee (1990-1995), for providing us with a quality product as the foundation for the revisions. The 2nd edition of the *Fetal Heart Monitoring Principles and Practices* book is built upon the framework and content of the 1st edition. The contributions of the content reviewers for both the 1st and 2nd editions also are acknowledged and appreciated.

2nd Edition Content Reviewers:	1st Edition Content Reviewers:
Donna Adelsperger, RNC, MEd	*Anne T. Barrett, RNC, MSN*
Julie Carr, RN, MSN	*Micki Cabaniss, MD*
Janet Cunningham, RNC, BSN, MS	*Catherine Driscoll, RN, BSN*
Deborah Davis, RNC, BSN	*Timothy R. B. Johnson, MD*
Michelle Murray, RNC, PhD	*Julian T. Parer, MD, PhD*
Anna Romig Nickels, RNC, BSN	*Jeffrey P. Phelan, MD, JD*
Julian T. Parer, MD, PhD	*Catherine C. Rommal, RNC, BS*
Jeffrey P. Phelan, MD, JD	*Kent Ueland, MD*
Judith Poole, RNC, MN	
Judy Schmidt, RNC, EdD	
Marie-Josée Trépanier, RNC, MEd	
Joyce Vogler, RN, Dr.PH, MS	
Faith Wight Moffatt, BN, MS (N)	

A special thanks also is extended to Patricia Wagner, RNC, MSN, innovator, contributor, member, and Chair of the Fetal Heart Monitoring Education Program Steering Committee from 1990 to 1991.

A special thanks also is extended to all of the AWHONN Fetal Heart Monitoring Principles and Practices Instructor Trainers and Instructors for their continuing support and participation.

A special thanks also is extended to Corometrics Medical Systems, Inc., for their generous contribution to support the revision of this resource book.

TABLE OF CONTENTS

PREFACE

The Fetal Heart Monitoring Principles and Practice Workshop (FHMPP) is a 2-day workshop (18.3 contact hours) focusing on the application of essential Fetal Heart Monitoring (FHM) knowledge and skills in nursing practice. The workshop is a method of validating a nurse's knowledge and skills to determine competence. The didactic session is an analysis of case studies that requires the synthesis of key principles pertinent to the physiologic basis of fetal heart monitoring technology, tracing interpretation, nursing intervention, and verbal and written communication skills. The skill sessions focus on demonstration and practice of skills, including auscultation, Leopold maneuvers, placing an intrauterine pressure catheter (IUPC) and spiral electrode, interpreting tracings, identifying indicated nursing interventions, and communication and documentation. Each section of the workshop builds upon principles addressed in the previous section. Successful completion of written exams and performance evaluations is a requirement for completion of the program and earning continuing education credit.

The FHMPP workshop is based on nursing and educational theory. The instructional design incorporates critical thinking and decision making and is specifically designed for professional nurses with previous FHM experience. Participants analyze multiple realistic case studies of increasing complexity and difficulty. Workshop participants are expected to have prior education and experience with both auscultation and EFM. Although the content of the workshop is comprehensive, specific nursing responsibilities vary according to institution, state, province, or region. Nurses who take the course are advised to be familiar with institutional policies and their state, province, or regional nurse practice act. Each institution must identify practice responsibilities as well as competence criteria and measurement.

Purpose: To validate the knowledge and skills of experienced nurses in a standardized FHM course.

Goal: To improve the assessment, promotion, and evaluation of fetal well being through dissemination of a standard course to validate the knowledge and skills of nurses whose practice includes FHR monitoring.

Objectives: Upon successful completion of the workshop, the participant will be able to

- Describe the role and responsibility of the professional nurse in the use of FHM.
- Demonstrate the necessary decision-making for the proper selection and verification of FHM techniques.
- Analyze FHR patterns and their implications for fetal well-being.
- Correlate indicated clinical interventions with related maternal-fetal physiology.
- Evaluate the fetal-maternal response to intervention.
- Simulate the psychomotor skills used in FHM.
- Communicate verbal and written data to verify accountability.

Content: The workshop applies principles of fetal heart monitoring to practice. The instructional methodology includes the manual, the didactic presentation, and the skill sessions.

1. Manual: The participant's resource manual reviews basic knowledge and skills used in FHM and is the companion text for the workshop. This manual is divided into chapters that correspond to the didactic case-study session topics and the nursing process (assessment, interpretation, intervention,

evaluation, and communication). Each chapter presents principles specific to that topic. The chapters review important areas of knowledge and skills and build upon the nurse's prior knowledge. Content includes a physiologic framework for decision making, contemporary technology, and complementary labor care. Professional standards of practice and clinical research are included with the discussion of practice principles. Additional chapters include a summary, a glossary, skill station outlines, and case-study exercises. This manual is intended to support the workshop objectives and is not intended to be a complete text of information for fetal heart monitoring practice.

2. Didactic: Didactic sessions present cognitive principles through case studies and include audiovisual and discussion methods. Actual case studies are used to provide practice-based discussion. Each case illustrates one or more specific principles or issues. Each section of the didactic portion builds upon the principles addressed in the scenarios of the previous section. Cases become successively more complex. The didactic discussion format allows participants to ask or respond to questions that help

- Extract key information.
- Identify the problem.
- Define the issues involved.
- Make decisions regarding appropriate nursing interventions.
- Evaluate outcome of interventions.
- Communicate and document the entire process.
- Formulate principles for handling future cases.

3. Skill Sessions: The hands-on skill sessions combine cognitive problem-solving simulations and psychomotor skills. The sessions include mechanisms for hands-on practice and validation of knowledge and skills using audiovisual and simulation models developed exclusively for the workshop. The skill sessions include

- Auscultation in FHM.
- Abdominal palpation in FHM.
- Instrumentation: Fetal spiral electrode and IUPC placement.
- Integration of FHM knowledge and skills through systematic strip interpretation (assessment, interpretation, intervention, and evaluation).
- Communication of FHM data.

Instruction and Administration:

For information regarding the AWHONN FHMPP workshop or other AWHONN workshop resources, please visit our website at http://www.awhonn.org, access AWHONN's Fax-on-Demand service by calling (800) 395-7373, or telephone headquarters at (800) 673-8499 if calling from the United States and (800) 245-0231 if calling from Canada.

Scheduling of workshops and preparation of instructors is conducted through this office. A portion of the workshop fee supports the many administration expenses, including staff support, design and production of course materials, distribution of materials, and committee activity.

CHAPTER 1: INTRODUCTION

The Association of Women's Health, Obstetric and Neonatal Nurses' (AWHONN) Fetal Heart Monitoring Principles and Practices (FHMPP) Workshop is an educational program for experienced professional nurses that provides both cognitive and psychomotor skill validation of standardized core competencies used in auscultation and electronic monitoring of the fetal heart rate (FHR). Workshop content is based on contemporary issues, current professional standards and research findings. Content includes fetal heart rate assessment as a component of individualized, comprehensive nursing care. Content is focused on intrapartum FHR monitoring; however, the knowledge and skills also are applied to FHR assessment in the antepartum period. Workshop methodology includes case studies, small group discussion, and simulated skill sessions. Chapter 1 includes a brief history of fetal heart rate monitoring practice and education and an overview of the FHMPP workshop. This edition includes feedback from many AWHONN FHMPP instructor-trainers, instructors, and past participants.

History of Fetal Heart Monitoring Practice

This brief history of fetal heart monitoring (FHM) practice provides a context for understanding the role of FHM in professional perinatal care. A more comprehensive historical review is found in the references and bibliography. A chronology of FHM developments is in Appendix 1a.

The evolution of FHM techniques was shaped by clinicians and researchers seeking ways to prevent fetal deaths. Contemporary FHM is the result of more than a century of research and development dedicated to improving obstetric care. Early practices in FHM were primitive compared with today's technology. Obstetric health care was complicated by issues as basic as whether a male physician should be permitted to touch or see an unclothed woman. The fetus was not recognized as a separate entity that could be included in the obstetric assessment until the 18th century. Interest in the fetus at that time focused on the recognition of fetal movement and the splashing sounds of the amniotic fluid (Goodlin, 1979).

An interest in fetal heart sounds developed nearly a century later with the almost simultaneous reports of the Swiss physician Mayor in 1818 and the French physician and nobleman Kergaradec in 1821. Both reported the presence of fetal heart sounds obtained by auscultation. Kergaradec used a stethoscope rather than the ear-to-abdomen method and is credited with being the first to recommend using fetal heart sounds for diagnostic purposes. In 1833, Kennedy of Dublin followed with a comprehensive monograph dedicated to convincing colleagues of the value of Kergaradec's technique of auscultating fetal heart sounds (Goodlin, 1979). The decades of the mid 19th century were notable for the variety of investigations on auscultated FHR data. Numerous reports defining the normal ranges of the FHR were published. These reports included correlating FHR information with maternal fever, fetal movement, gestational age, fetal weight, and fetal sex. Frankenhauser reported that female fetuses demonstrated a higher average heart rate (144 beats per minute) than males (124 beats per minute), which was undoubtedly the origin of the still common myth (Wulf, 1985).

1

Throughout the 19th century, clinicians debated methods of auscultation (stethoscope versus ear-to-abdomen), the positioning of the patient (standing versus supine), and the necessity of baring the pregnant abdomen during the procedure. Late in the 19th century, several physicians recognized the clinical significance of repeated auscultation of fetal heart sounds during labor. In Germany, Schwartz suggested that the FHR be counted often during labor, between and during contractions, as a method of assessing fetal well-being. His 1858 text presented a concept of asphyxia associated with the first breath and related fetal bradycardia to decreased placental function caused by the reduction in blood flow during contractions. Schwartz is credited with being the first to investigate fetal breathing activity. Numerous other investigators joined the search for the pathophysiology underlying FHR changes. By the end of the century, the impact of head and cord compression and uterine activities on FHR findings was recognized. In 1888, Killian, an American, was credited with being the first to propose that FHR information be used to identify the need for intervening in fetal distress. One year later, in Germany, Winckel described specific criteria to be used in diagnosing fetal distress by FHR auscultation. Winckel's criteria were accepted without reservation until 1958, when Hon raised serious concerns over the subjectivity of human counting of fetal heart sounds.

Use of technology in FHM began early in the 20th century with Cremer's use of abdominal and vaginal electrodes to obtain a fetal electrocardiogram. By the 1950s, research on electronic methods of FHM escalated because of growing doubts about the validity of FHR data obtained intermittently by auscultation for predicting fetal well-being and planning intervention. By the 1960s, Hon, Caldeyro-Barcia, and Hammacher were reporting successful attempts at developing an electronic FHR monitor that could continuously record FHR information (Caldeyro-Barcia & Mendez-Bauer, 1966; Hammacher, 1969; Hon, 1963). At the same time, these researchers were investigating patterns of FHR responses to various events and circumstances and associated physiologic mechanisms. During the 1970s, electronic fetal monitoring (EFM) with sophisticated equipment was introduced into widespread use in obstetric care.

Throughout the century preceding the introduction of electronic FHM, the value of uterine activity monitoring during labor was examined. In 1872, Schatz placed balloons within the uterus to record intrauterine pressures. Two decades later, Schaffer attempted to obtain uterine activity data externally through use of a hood and an attached spirometer placed over the pregnant abdomen. These early attempts to monitor uterine contractions went beyond attempts to define normal values, as investigators also studied the uterine response to anesthetics and drugs, such as epinephrine, ether, and morphine (Goodlin, 1979).

During the post-World War II decade, new devices were developed that provided the basis for EFM technology. The tocodynamometer, an external device to continuously detect a close approximation of the frequency, duration, and relative strength of uterine contractions was introduced. The introduction of this device was soon followed by the development of a device to measure intrauterine pressure. A catheter could be inserted through the cervix and attached to an external strain gauge transducer to record intrauterine pressure. Post-war research also led to medical use of Doppler ultrasound technology. This technology provided the basis for the external method of continuously recording FHR that was to be introduced two decades later.

The definitions related to FHR patterns are based on the findings of Caldeyro-Barcia and Mendez-Bauer; Hammacher; and Hon. During the 1950s and 1960s, these physicians studied and defined the baseline rate according to oscillation characteristics. Alterations in the baseline rate were described as an acceleration or deceleration in the FHR (Table 1-1). Variability was described as irregularities of the baseline FHR and classified by the amplitude of the FHR fluctuations and the number of cycle changes per minute (Hon, 1963). Caldeyro-Barcia and Mendez-Bauer (1966) described variability as rapid fluctuations with an amplitude range of 1-8 beats per minute with 3-10 cycles per minute. Hammacher, Huter, and Bokelmann (1968) were the first to attribute clinical significance to short-term or beat-to-beat variability. Hon and Caldeyro-Barcia and Mendez-Bauer agreed upon their descriptions of FHR patterns, but Hon's actual definitions formed the basis of pattern description. Discrepant categories of variability have evolved. There has never been a consensus on which category of variability should be used (Table 1-2). Disagreement continues among researchers and practitioners regarding description of FHR changes, terminology, and interpretation.

In 1995, the National Institute of Child Health and Human Development (NICHD) at the National Institutes of Health (NIH) brought together an international panel of experts whose mission was to develop standard definitions of EFM patterns for use in research. Research using standard definitions will facilitate measurement of the predictive value of EFM and thus contribute to evidence-based practice (Harvey & Chez, 1996). At this printing, the consensus has not been reported.

Hon (1963)	Caldeyro-Barcia and Mendez-Bauer (1966)	Hammacher (1969)
baseline irregularity	bradycardia	type 0 oscillation silent pattern
bradycardia	tachycardia	type 1 oscillations narrow undulating
tachycardia	type I dip	type 2 oscillations undulating pattern
early deceleration	type II dip	type 0 dip
late deceleration	baseline rapid fluctuation	type 1 dip
variable deceleration	transient ascents of FHR	type 2 dip

Table 1-1. Historical Classifications of Fetal Heart Rate and Variability

Levels of Categorization	Categories of Variability Nomenclature			
	V	IV	III	II
0-2 bpm	Absent	Absent	Decreased	Absent
3-5 bpm	Minimal	Minimal		
6-15 bpm	Average	Average	Average	Present
15-25 bpm	Moderate			
>25 bpm	Marked	Marked	Increased	

Table 1-2. Categories of Variability Nomenclature (Adapted from Chez & Harvey, 1994)

The introduction of electronic FHM as a method of assessing fetal well-being during labor altered obstetric practice. In many settings electronic monitoring quickly evolved into the primary technique for FHM, with auscultation used as a screening or secondary technique. In some settings, intermittent auscultation continued to be used.

Professional organizations began to incorporate fetal heart monitoring responsibilities, both auscultation and electronic, into existing practice policy statements and resources (Table 1-3). For example, AWHONN, formerly The Nurses Association of the American College of Obstetricians and Gynecologists (NAACOG), has provided competence guidelines, position statements, and standards for fetal heart monitoring nursing practice. These resources are revised on the basis of new research findings, and technological advances.

At the same time that electronic monitoring was being introduced, other dimensions of obstetric practice were being revised in a continuing effort to reduce perinatal morbidity and mortality. As the cost and invasiveness of many aspects of obstetric care escalated, consumers and professionals questioned universal use of EFM. Early investigations that attempted to validate the efficacy of modern technology over auscultation were confounded by design and patient selection factors. New guidelines for FHR assessment during labor were published (American College of Obstetricians and Gynecologists [ACOG], 1987; NAACOG, 1990). Research on the safety and efficacy of EFM continued (Thacker, Stroup, & Peterson, 1995) and in 1995 ACOG stated "current data indicate that FHR monitoring is equally effective whether done electronically or by auscultation" (ACOG, 1995). The Society of Obstetricians and Gynecologists of Canada (SOGC) stated that intermittent auscultation is the recommended method of FHR surveillance for low risk women during labor (SOGC, 1995). The use of EFM in low-risk births has been challenged in the nursing literature (Supplee & Vezeau, 1996). Even with these position statements and guidelines, differences of opinions remain regarding choice of monitoring method, terminology, pattern definitions and significance, and impact on patient management.

Source	Year	Title
NAACOG	1990	*Fetal Heart Rate Auscultation.* OGN Nursing Practice Resource.
NAACOG	1991	*Nursing Practice Competencies and Educational Guidelines: Antepartum Fetal Surveillance and Intrapartum Fetal Heart Monitoring (2nd ed.).* Guidelines.
NAACOG	1991	*NAACOG Standards for the Nursing Care of Women and Newborns (4th ed.).*
ACNM	1991	*Appropriate Use of Technology in Childbirth.* Position Statement.
AWHONN	1992	*Nursing Responsibilities in Implementing Fetal Heart Rate Monitoring.* Position Statement.
AAP & ACOG	1992	*Antepartum and Intrapartum Care. Guidelines for Perinatal Care (3rd ed.).* Guidelines.
AWHONN	1993	*Didactic Content and Clinical Skills Verification for Professional Nurse Providers of Basic, High Risk and Critical Care Intrapartum Nursing.* Guidelines.
SOGC	1995	*Fetal Health Surveillance in Labor.* SOGC Policy Statement.
ACOG	1995	*Fetal Heart Rate Patterns: Monitoring, Interpretation and Management.* ACOG Technical Bulletin No. 207.

Table 1-3. Professional Standards for Fetal Heart Monitoring

Table Legend

NAACOG - The Nurses Association of the American College of Obstetricians and Gynecologists
ACNM - The American College of Nurse Midwives
AAP - The American Academy of Pediatrics
ACOG - The American College of Obstetricians and Gynecologists
AWHONN - The Association of Women's Health, Obstetric and Neonatal Nurses (formerly NAACOG)
SOGC - The Society of Obstetricians and Gynaecologists of Canada

---

Historically, the goal of fetal heart monitoring was to identify FHR changes that indicated a fetus at risk for asphyxia. After more than two decades of research and experience using electronic FHM, considerable information exists about the nature and implications of alterations in the FHR. As this knowledge base has expanded, so has the recognition that reassuring and favorable findings can be equally helpful in providing care to the maternal-fetal unit. The purpose of fetal heart monitoring is now believed to be both identification of the fetus experiencing well-being and the fetus experiencing compromise.

History of Fetal Heart Rate Monitoring Education

Physicians and midwives used auscultation of fetal heart sounds as a method of assessing fetal well-being as early as the beginning of the 19th century. Electronic FHM technology has been used for this purpose for more than two decades now. Although fetal monitoring often is equated with electronic technology, both electronic and nonelectronic methods are used to assess FHR and uterine activity, and caregivers interpret data gathered by both manual and technological methods. Fetal heart monitoring education programs should help health care providers develop critical thinking and decision-making skills, including synthesizing and evaluating data from several sources. Competence in fetal monitoring requires maternal-fetal physiology knowledge, interpretation and decision-making skills, and psychomotor skills.

When electronic FHM was introduced, formal education in the technique was either nonexistent or provided by the consumer services divisions of equipment manufacturers. Most nurses trained in FHM during this era learned basic application of the new technology through on-the-job experience alone. Gradually, researchers and clinicians developed electronic FHM education programs and provided these across the country. This informal network of independent FHM educators was, and continues to be, a primary source of FHM instruction. Programs also were developed to train instructors in the knowledge and skills necessary for teaching basic FHM (Adelsperger, 1990; Traber, Leppein, & Billmaier, 1993). The continuing contribution of the many nurse-experts who develop EFM education programs must be acknowledged. These nurses provide a valuable source for continuing education and their programs were, and continue to be, important in the dissemination of basic and advanced electronic FHM knowledge and skills.

Textbooks in medicine and nursing began to include basic instruction on the nature and purpose of this new technology early in the history of EFM. However, student instruction on EFM tends to be limited to brief lectures and clinical rotations in the labor and delivery unit. New nurse graduates often do not have basic skills in fetal heart monitoring, either auscultation or electronic.

The professional organizations, including AWHONN and ACOG, began to provide educational resources as EFM was integrated into practice. Technical bulletins and practice resources were published as practice standards developed. In 1977, ACOG produced a slide-tape module on the basics of electronic FHM which was widely used in hospital inservice programs.

By the early 1980s, the emphasis, style, and content of education in electronic FHM was quite diverse. Clinicians repeatedly sought resources for two central tasks: identifying aspects of EFM that are core to competent practice and establishing mechanisms for validating appropriate knowledge and skill. Professional competence guidelines and educational materials were developed to address these tasks.

In the mid 1980s, NAACOG convened a national task force of nurse experts to establish a framework to address these issues. In 1986, this task force published the handbook Electronic Fetal Monitoring: Nursing Practice Competencies and Educational Guidelines (NAACOG, 1986), which was later updated as Nursing Practice Competencies and Educational Guidelines: Antepartum Fetal Surveillance and Intrapartum Fetal Heart Monitoring (NAACOG, 1991b). These competence guidelines state that educational programs should include both core (basic) and ongoing (experienced) instructional programs. A core program includes essential knowledge and skills to achieve minimal competence, while an ongoing experienced program includes additional knowledge and skills to maintain competence. The guidelines specify that evaluation techniques may include such activities as examination, case-study analysis, tracing interpretation, role-play, policy and documentation discussion, and skill demonstration. In addition to regular revision of the competence guidelines, guidelines for general nursing care and resources for competence validation have been developed (AWHONN, 1993; NAACOG, 1991a) (Table 1-3).

In 1988, NAACOG produced a videotape series titled Essentials of Electronic Fetal Heart Monitoring for both basic instruction and knowledge validation (Chez & Murray, 1988) and a text titled Antepartal & Intrapartal Fetal Monitoring for basic and advanced information (Murray, 1988). A continued demand for electronic FHM practice resources led to a second module of five videotapes, collectively titled Critical Concepts in Fetal Heart Rate Monitoring (Chez, Harvey, & Murray, 1989), which was updated in 1996 (Harvey & Chez, 1996). These video programs included content on issues, such as equipment troubleshooting and fetal blood sampling. A resource manual to help health care professionals develop FHM policies, procedures, protocols, and documentation formats also was developed to accompany the videotape series. These resources continue to be updated by AWHONN.

In 1987, ACOG published guidelines for FHM during labor, which reaffirmed the technique of auscultation as a primary intrapartum nursing skill and as an important component in EFM (ACOG, 1987). In 1990, NAACOG produced the practice resource Fetal Heart Rate Auscultation, which included physiologic principles, terminology, techniques, interpretation, and documentation (NAACOG, 1990). Palpation of both uterine activity and fetal presentation and position using Leopold's maneuvers received renewed attention as a primary skill in the appropriate use of both techniques of FHM.

NAACOG began the second phase of its electronic FHM educational effort in 1990 by planning a standardized course for validation of core concepts in the use of auscultation and EFM. The focus on skills validation in many areas of nursing practice had increased, leading to the development of new models of continuing nurse education.

The NAACOG Committee on Education appointed a National Steering Committee of nurse experts in fetal monitoring education. This committee was to develop a course that would apply concepts to practice through the use of small group, case study, and hands-on instructional methods. This course would complement institutional programs on basic monitoring knowledge and skills. A 2-day course was created including development of a workshop manual, audiovisual materials, and models. The plan included training qualified NAACOG members as course instructors to teach the course and as course instructor-trainers to prepare additional instructors. Since 1993, the original instructor-trainers have continued to prepare qualified nurses as course instructors to teach the Fetal Heart Monitoring Principles & Practices (FHMPP) workshop. The Instructor Enhancement Course was developed in 1994 to provide further support for developing course instructors. At the end of 1996, there were more than 650 FHMPP instructors located throughout the United States and abroad. More than 900 FHMPP workshops have been conducted since 1993, with more than 10,000 participants, in the United States, Canada, Germany, Italy, Spain, and Turkey. A newsletter, *The Beat Goes On*, was developed to update both course instructors and instructor-trainers on program changes.

Several issues regarding fetal heart monitoring competency validation have been addressed in the literature (Afriat, Simpson, Chez, & Miller, 1994). During development of the FHMPP education program, the topic of whether nurses should obtain credentialing or certification in fetal heart monitoring arose. Central issues that surrounded the discussion included the following:

- Standards of national accreditation organizations (such as the Joint Commission on Accreditation of Health Care Organizations) which require core competence validations.

- Limitations for standardization because of experts' lack of consensus on terminology and interpretation.

- Adaptation of instruction and evaluation to the novice and experienced nurse.

- Numerous methods of verifying competence.

- Individual institutional needs.

- The relationship of fetal monitoring competence to a comprehensive maternal-fetal nursing care competence validation program.

AWHONN decided to provide the FHMPP workshop as a complement to the existing AWHONN resources on basic fetal heart monitoring. The program is designed to validate the cognitive knowledge and skills of the experienced nurse in comprehensive fetal heart monitoring (auscultation and electronic fetal heart monitoring). Fetal monitoring is placed within the nursing model, as a component of overall nursing knowledge and skills, and not as an isolated technical skill. The FHMPP workshop was designed to be part of an overall plan for competence validation in specialty practice for the institution or individual. Many jurisdictions and health organizations use the workshop for this purpose.

Even with the volume of FHM education occurring at this time, there is limited research examining practice, knowledge and skills, or education methods. Studies addressing nursing skill in fetal heart monitoring have included examining skill in categorizing electronic tracings (Chez et al., 1990) and testing feasibility of the auscultation method (Morrison et al., 1993; Paine, 1992). Recent investigation has addressed the capabilities of computerized analysis of electronic FHR patterns (Farmakides & Weiner, 1995). Some researchers have found performance of an "intelligent" computer system to be indistinguishable from expert physician clinicians, as measured by degree of agreement in labor management decisions based on interpretation of cardiotocograms (Keith et al., 1995). Studies addressing nursing education in FHM have examined skill expectations, instructional methodology, and knowledge and skill differences (Kinnick, 1989, 1990; McCartney, 1995; Murray, 1992; Sauer, 1993; Trepanier et al., 1996). Further studies are needed to guide FHM practice and education.

The Nursing Process and the FHMPP Education Program

The nursing process model provides the theoretical framework for the structure and process of this book and the FHMPP workshop. The content structure in this book and the didactic components of the workshop follow the standard phases of the nursing process (assessment, interpretation, intervention, and evaluation). The process of FHM decision-making is based on the critical-thinking skills of analysis, synthesis, and evaluation found in the nursing process (Figure 1-1).

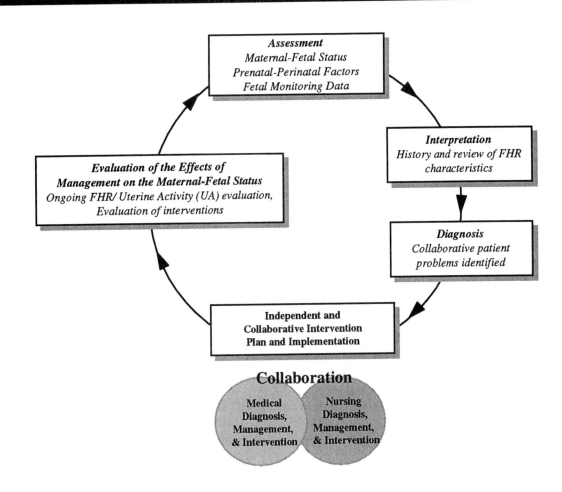

Figure 1-1. The Nursing Process and Fetal Heart Monitoring

The FHMPP education program also is based on problem-centered or case study education methodology aimed at helping learners understand specific problems encountered in the work setting (McDonald, 1990; Parker, 1990). Problem Based Learning (PBL) presents students with learning tasks similar to practice (often a written patient case) and focuses on the goal of application in practice rather than on accumulation of facts (Barrows & Tamblyn, 1980). Information in the case study is presented in segments, and students work in small groups to systematically assess, analyze, and interpret problem cues and to discuss intervention. Students are expected to build on prior knowledge, and faculty is expected to guide, stimulate, and foster critical thinking skills as well as present structured advanced information. Often, the integration of knowledge and skills is accomplished through skills training and practice. Methodologies, such as case studies, simulations, and discussions are believed to be effective for learning the practical knowledge and skills of clinical nursing (Benner, 1984). This method was selected to focus on clinical decision-making skills. Novice nurses' learning needs for context-free factual information are different from experienced nurses' learning needs for case studies, discussion, and reflection. Both education and experience are necessary to achieve the skilled clinical judgment of the expert professional nurse (Benner, 1984).

Instruction with case studies requires integrating fetal heart monitoring data, including technologically generated data, into a broader clinical assessment. As nurses use more technologically generated data there is a risk of technological dependency (Sandelowski, 1993). Aspects of technology dependency to consider in FHM education include reliance and emphasis on assessing data generated by technology and developing electronic monitoring skill at the expense of developing other assessment skills. Technology also requires the efficient investment of resources necessary for developing and maintaining electronic monitoring skills.

A complete description of the FHMPP workshop and information is included in the Preface.

APPENDIX 1a: A Condensed Chronology of FHM Developments

1818	Swiss surgeon, Mayor, reports hearing FHR by placing ear on patient's abdomen.
1821	French physician, Kergaradec, reports FHR obtained by stethoscope and is first to recognize value in diagnosing fetal life and well-being.
1833	Irish physician, Kennedy, publishes comprehensive monograph describing patterns of the FHR and emphasizing the value of Kergaradec's technique.
1858	Schwartz publishes first investigation of fetal breathing activity and its relationship to FHR and placental sufficiency.
1860	Frankenhauser reports study of influencing factors, including sex differences in average FHRs.
1872	Schatz places balloons within the uterus to record intrauterine pressures.
1888	Kilian becomes first to propose that FHR be used to diagnose need for intervention for fetal distress.
1889	Winckel publishes an obstetric textbook that identifies specific criteria for diagnosing fetal distress by auscultation. These criteria are used until the 1960s.
1896	Schäeffer reports attempts to measure uterine activity by using an externally placed device attached to spirometer.
1906	Cremer reports on the fetal electrocardiogram (ECG) for the first time using abdominal and intravaginal leads.
1908	Wasenius reports use of Schatz techniques to study the effects of ether and morphine upon uterine contractions.
1947	Reynolds develops a multichannel tocodynamometer capable of making uterine tension measurements.
1952	Williams and Stallworthy report use of a polyethylene catheter placed through the cervix of a laboring patient to record intrauterine pressure and become some of the first to relate uterine activity to fetal well-being.
1952	Caldeyro-Barcia develops formula for measuring uterine pressures and defines "Montevideo Unit" to quantify uterine activity.
1958	Hon provides a preliminary report on FHM research.
1960s	Hon in America, Caldeyro-Barcia in Uruguay, and Hammacher in Germany publish pioneer FHM research.
1961	Saling performs first measurement of fetal pH.
1963	Hon modifies the Michelle Skin Clip, known as the clip electrode, to monitor the FHR directly.
1964	Callagan et al. describe a practical Doppler ultrasound instrument that can be used to detect human heart sound: 2 years later, use of the device in FHR detection is reported.
1967	Hon and Caldeyro-Barcia establish definitions of FHR patterns to be used in fetal monitoring.
1970s	Real-time ultrasound begins.
1970s	Fetal scalp and umbilical acid-base technique incorporated into practice.
1970s	A contraction stress test is developed.
1971	Hon and Caldeyro-Barcia collaborate to standardize terminology from Caldeyro-Barcia's Type I and Type II to Hon's earlys, lates, and variables.
1972	Hon develops the spiral electrode.
1976	A nonstress test is developed.
1977	Read and Miller use fetal acoustic stimulation.
1980	Doppler flow studies begin.
1980s	A biophysical profile is developed.
1980s	Sensor-tipped catheter is introduced (also called solid-state).
1983	Second-generation monitors that use autocorrelation are introduced.
1989	Home uterine monitoring is introduced.
1990	Twin ultrasound monitor is introduced.
1991	A monitor that detects fetal movement and duplicates heartbeat of one twin is introduced.

REFERENCES

Adelsperger, D. (1990). Train the trainer program. Continuing Education Program. Washington, DC: AWHONN.

Afriat, C., Simpson, K., Chez, B., & Miller, L. (1994). Electronic fetal monitoring competency—To validate or not to validate: The opinions of experts. Journal of Perinatal and Neonatal Nursing, 8(3), 1-16.

American Academy of Pediatrics and American College of Obstetricians and Gynecologists (AAP & ACOG). (1992). Guidelines for Perinatal Care (3rd ed.). Elk Grove Village, IL: Author.

American College of Nurse Midwives (ACNM). (1991). The appropriate use of technology in childbirth. Position Statement. Washington, DC: Author.

American College of Obstetricians and Gynecologists (ACOG). (1987). Standards for obstetric—gynecologic services (6th ed.). Washington, DC: Author.

American College of Obstetricians and Gynecologists (ACOG). (1995). Fetal heart rate patterns: Monitoring, interpretation, and management. ACOG Technical Bulletin No. 207. Washington, DC: Author.

Association of Women's Health, Obstetric and Neonatal Nurses (AWHONN). (1992). Nursing responsibilities in implementing intrapartum fetal heart rate monitoring. Position Statement. Washington, DC: Author.

Association of Women's Health, Obstetric and Neonatal Nurses (AWHONN). (1993). Didactic content and clinical skills verification for professional nurse providers of basic, high risk, and critical care intrapartum nursing. Washington, DC: Author.

Barrows, H.S., & Tamblyn, R.M. (1980). Problem based learning: An approach to medical education. New York: Springer.

Benner, P. (1984). From novice to expert: Excellence and power in clinical nursing practice. Menlo Park, CA: Addison-Wesley.

Caldeyro-Barcia, R., Mendez-Bauer, E., & Poseiro, J. (1966). Control of human fetal heart rate during labor. In D. E. Cassels (Ed.), The heart and circulation in the newborn and infant (p. 7). New York: Grune and Stratton.

Chez, B. F., & Murray, M. (1988). Essentials of electronic fetal heart monitoring. Videotape series: Nurses Association of the American College of Obstetricians and Gynecologists (NAACOG). Baltimore, MD: Williams and Wilkins.

Chez, B. F., Harvey, C., & Murray, M. (1989). Critical concepts in fetal heart rate monitoring. Videotape series: Nurses Association of the American College of Obstetricians and Gynecologists (NAACOG). Baltimore, MD: Williams and Wilkins.

Chez, B. F., & Harvey, C. (1994). Essentials of electronic fetal heart monitoring (2nd ed.). Videotape series: Association of Women's Health, Obstetric and Neonatal Nurses (AWHONN). Baltimore, MD: Williams and Wilkins.

Chez, B., Skurnick, J., Chez, R., Verklan, M., Biggs, S., & Hage, M. (1990). Interpretations of nonstress tests by obstetric nurses. Journal of Obstetric, Gynecologic, and Neonatal Nurses, 19(3), 227-233.

Farmakides, G., & Weiner, Z. (1995). Computerized analysis of the fetal heart rate. Clinical Obstetrics and Gynecology, 38(1), 112-120.

Goodlin, R. C. (1979). History of fetal monitoring. American Journal of Obstetrics and Gynecology, 133, 323-352.

Hammacher, K., Huter, K., & Bokelmann, J. (1968). Foetal heart frequency and perinatal condition of the foetus and newborn. Gynaecologia, 166, 349.

Hammacher, K. (1969). The clinical significance of cardiotocography. In P. Huntingford, K. Huter, & E. Salez (Eds.), Perinatal medicine, 1st European Congress, Berlin, (p.81). New York: Academic Press.

Harvey, C., & Chez, B. F. (1996). Critical concepts in fetal heart rate monitoring (2nd ed.). Videotape series: Association of Women's Health, Obstetric and Neonatal Nurses (AWHONN). Baltimore, MD: Williams and Wilkins.

Hon, E. (1963). The classification of fetal heart rate: A revised working classification. Obstetrics and Gynecology, 22, 137.

Keith, R., Beckley, S., Garibaldi, J., Westgate, J., Ifeachor, E., & Greene, K. (1995). A multicentre comparative study of 17 experts and an intelligent computer system for managing labour using the cardiotocogram. British Journal of Obstetrics and Gynecology, 102(9), 688-700.

Kinnick, V.G. (1989). A national survey about fetal monitoring skills acquired by nursing students in baccalaureate programs. Journal of Obstetric, Gynecologic, and Neonatal Nurses (JOGNN), 18(1), 57-58.

Kinnick, V.G. (1990). The effect of concept teaching in preparing nursing students for clinical practice. Journal of Nursing Education, 29(8), 362-366.

McCartney, P. (1995). Fetal heart rate pattern analysis by expert and novice nurses. Dissertation Abstracts International. 56-07, Section B, 3677-3944. Unpublished doctoral dissertation. (University Microfilms No. 9538106).

McDonald, B. A. (1990, August). Begin course development with a course blueprint. Performance and Instruction, 29(10), 4.

Morrison, J., Chez, B., Davis, I., Martin, R., Roberts, W., Martin, J., & Floyd, R. (1993). Intrapartum fetal heart rate assessment: Monitoring by auscultation or electronic means. American Journal of Obstetrics and Gynecology, 168(1), 63-66.

Murray, M. (1988). Antepartal and intrapartal fetal monitoring. Washington, DC: NAACOG.

Murray, M. L. (1992). A comparison of fetal monitoring concept learning from a learner-controlled versus teacher-controlled instructional strategy. Unpublished doctoral dissertation, University of New Mexico, Albuquerque, NM.

Nurses Association of the American College of Obstetricians and Gynecologists (NAACOG). (1986). Nursing practice competencies and educational guidelines. Washington, DC: Author.

Nurses Association of the American College of Obstetricians and Gynecologists (NAACOG). (1990). Fetal heart rate auscultation, OGN Nursing Practice Resource. Washington, DC: Author.

Nurses Association of the American College of Obstetricians and Gynecologists (NAACOG). (1991a). Competency validation (2nd ed.). Washington, DC: Author.

Nurses Association of the American College of Obstetricians and Gynecologists (NAACOG). (1991b). Nursing practice competencies and educational guidelines: Antepartum fetal surveillance and intrapartum fetal heart monitoring (2nd ed.). Washington, DC: Author.

Paine, L. (1992). A comparison of the auscultated acceleration test and the nonstress test as predictors of perinatal outcomes. Nursing Research, 41(2), 87-91.

Parker, E. T. (1990). Back to Socrates: Problem-centered course design. Performance and Instruction, 29(10), 47.

Sandelowski, M. (1993). Toward a theory of technological dependency. Nursing Outlook, 41(1), 36-42.

Sauer, P. (1993, June). Interpretations of fetal heart rate tracings by obstetric nurses: Comparison of test scores with experience and education in electronic fetal heart rate monitoring. Poster session presented at the annual meeting of the Association of Women's Health, Obstetric and Neonatal Nurses, Reno, NV.

Society of Obstetricians and Gynaecologists of Canada (SOGC). (1995). SOGC Policy Statement: Fetal health surveillance in labour. Journal of SOGC, 17(9), 865-901.

Supplee, R. B., & Vezeau, T. M. (1996). Continuous electronic fetal monitoring: Does it belong in low-risk births? Maternal Child Nursing, 21, 301-306.

Thacker, S.B., Stroup, D.F., & Peterson, H.B. (1995). Efficacy and Safety of Intrapartum Electronic Fetal Monitoring: An Update. Obstetrics and Gynecology, 86(4), 613-620.

Traber, E., Leppein, M., & Billmaier, K. (1993, June). Development of a regional EFM train the trainer program. Poster session presented at the annual meeting of the Association of Women's Health, Obstetric and Neonatal Nurses, Reno, NV.

Trepanier, M., Niday, P., Davies, B., Sprague, A., Nimrod, C., Dulberg, C., & Watters, N. (1996). Evaluation of a fetal monitoring education program. Journal of Obstetric, Gynecologic, and Neonatal Nurses, 25(2), 137-144.

Wulf, K. H. (1985). History of fetal heart rate monitoring. In W. Kunzel (Ed.), <u>Fetal heart rate monitoring</u> (p. 3-19). New York: Springer-Verlag.

BIBLIOGRAPHY

Afriat, C., & Schifrin, B. S. (1976). Sources of error in fetal heart rate monitoring. <u>Journal of Obstetric, Gynecologic, and Neonatal Nursing, 5</u>(Suppl. 5), 11-15.

Afriat, C. (1987). Historical perspectives on electronic fetal heart rate monitoring: A decade of growth, a decade of conflict. <u>Journal of Perinatal Neonatal Nursing, 5</u>(Suppl. 5), 1-4.

Blackburn, S., & Loper, D. (1992). <u>Maternal fetal and neonatal physiology</u>. New York: W.B. Saunders.

Chagnon, L., & Easterwood, B. (1986). Managing the risks of obstetrical nursing. <u>American Journal of Maternal Child Nursing, 11</u>, 303-310.

Eliason, M. J., & Williams, J. K. (1990). Fetal alcohol syndrome and the neonate. <u>Journal of Perinatal Neonatal Nursing, 3</u>(4), 64-72.

Ettinger, B., & McCart, D. (1976). Effects of drugs on the FHR during labor. <u>Journal of Obstetric, Gynecologic, and Neonatal Nursing, 5</u>(Suppl. 5), 41-51.

Fields, L. (1987). Electronic fetal monitoring: Practice and protocols for the intrapartum patient. <u>Journal of Perinatal Neonatal Nursing, 1</u>(1), 5-12.

Freeman, R. K., Gutterrez, N. A., Ray, M. L., Stovall, D., Paul, R. H., & Hon, E. H. (1972). Fetal cardiac response to paracervical block anesthesia. Part 1. <u>American Journal of Obstetrics and Gynecology, 113</u>, 583-591.

Freeman, R. K., Garite, T. J., & Nageotte, M. P. (1991). (2nd ed.). <u>Fetal heart rate monitoring</u>. Baltimore: Williams and Wilkins.

Freinkel, N. (Ed.). (1985). Summary and recommendations of the Second International Workshop Conference on Gestational Diabetes Mellitus. <u>Diabetes, 34</u>(Suppl.), 123-126.

Gabbe, S. (1986). Definition, detection, and management of gestational diabetes. <u>Obstetrics and Gynecology, 67</u>(1), 121-125.

Havercamp, A. D., & Cetrulo, C. (1976). The evaluation of continuous fetal heart rate monitoring in high risk pregnancy. <u>American Journal of Obstetrics and Gynecology, 125</u>, 310.

Kennard, M. J. (1990). Cocaine use during pregnancy: Fetal and neonatal effects. <u>Journal of Perinatal Neonatal Nursing, 3</u>(4), 53-63.

Kuller, J. M. (1990). Effects on the fetus and newborn of medications commonly used during pregnancy. <u>Journal of Perinatal Neonatal Nursing, 3</u>(4), 73-87.

Martin, C. B., & Gingerich, B. (1976). Uteroplacental physiology. <u>Journal of Obstetric, Gynecologic, and Neonatal Nursing, 5</u>(Suppl. 5), 16-24.

Martin, C. B., & Gingerich, B. (1976). Factors affecting the fetal heart rate: Genesis of fetal heart rate patterns. <u>Journal of Obstetric, Gynecologic, and Neonatal Nursing, 5</u> (Suppl. 5), 30-40.

Martin, C. B. (1982). Physiology and clinical use of fetal heart rate variability. <u>Clinics in Perinatology,</u> <u>9</u>(2), 339-352.

Moore, M. L. (1983). <u>Realities in childbearing</u> (2nd ed.). Philadelphia: W. B. Saunders Company.

Murray, M.L. (1997). <u>Antepartal & Intrapartal Fetal Monitoring</u> (2nd ed.). Albuquerque, NM: Learning Resources International.

Parer, J. T. (1983). <u>Handbook of fetal heart rate monitoring</u>. Philadelphia: W.B. Saunders.

Parer, J. T. (1994). Fetal heart rate. In R. K. Creasy & R. Resnik (Eds.), <u>Maternal fetal medicine:</u> <u>Principle and practices</u> (3rd ed.). Philadelphia: W. B. Saunders Company.

Peley, D. (1979). FHR Patterns: Study of anencephalic infants. <u>Obstetrics and Gynecology, 53</u>, 530.

Poole, J. (1988). Getting perspective on HELLP syndrome. <u>Maternal Child Nursing, 13</u>, 432-437.

Prichard, J. A., MacDonald, R. C., & Gant, N. F. (1985). <u>Williams Obstetrics</u> (20th ed). Norwalk, CT: Appleton & Lange.

Schifrin, B. (1990). <u>Exercises in fetal monitoring</u>. St. Louis: Mosby Year Book.

Wiley, J. (1976). The nurse's legal responsibility in obstetrical monitoring. <u>Journal of Obstetric,</u> <u>Gynecologic, and Neonatal Nursing, 5</u>(Suppl. 5), 77-78.

CHAPTER 2: ASSESSMENT: NURSING DATA BASE

Introduction

This chapter reviews the critical concepts for the nursing process assessment of the perinatal patient, specifically related to fetal well-being (Figure 2-1). A comprehensive assessment includes the maternal-fetal status, perinatal factors, and fetal monitoring data. This chapter outlines the physiologic basis of the FHR response and introduces the Dynamic Physiologic Response Model (Figure 2-10) for conceptualizing this physiologic basis. This chapter also outlines the techniques and instrumentation of FHM. Application of the nursing process provides a consistent, logical framework for practice and directs the problem-solving process. The standard nursing steps of assessment, interpretation, planning, intervention and evaluation furnish a structure for organizing and responding to individual patient situations.

To perform the steps of assessment and determine a specific maternal-fetal dyad's nursing needs, a complete nursing data base on the family is assembled. This data base includes historical data (prenatal and preconception history, admission interview data) as well as information on current physiological status of the mother and fetus (maternal-fetal physical assessment). This information is then continuously updated and simultaneously analyzed, to identify problems or potential problems that put the mother and/or fetus at risk of adverse outcomes or to provide reassurance of maternal and fetal well-being.

However, data alone will not provide perinatal caregivers with an accurate understanding of maternal-fetal status. It is important to understand the maternal-fetal anatomy, physiologic processes and the clinical significance of the data to formulate a complete assessment. In addition, knowledge about the benefits and limitations of each monitoring method and the data produced is needed. The analysis of any type of data, whether from auscultation of the heart rate, EFM, vital signs, or maternal history, can only prove meaningful when the practitioner involved understands the physiologic significance of the data within the individual clinical situation.

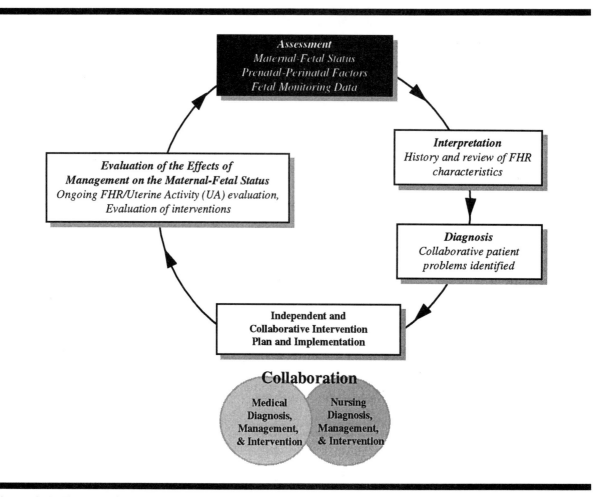

Figure 2-1. The nursing process and fetal heart monitoring: Assessment

<u>Maternal-Fetal Historical Data</u>

The review of prenatal records and the admission interview provide historical data on the maternal-fetal dyad (Figure 2-1). This data has many uses; however, the focus will be on the implications for fetal surveillance during the intrapartum period.

By reviewing the information obtained from the patient's history, it may be possible to identify the presence of risk factors that may increase the risk of complications in the perinatal period. While the presence of risk factors is not predictive of outcomes, an awareness of risk factors may be helpful in understanding fetal physiologic responses during this period. A list of many variables identified as risk factors is provided (Appendix 2a). While risk assessment tools have been tested, no tool is currently available that can accurately predict and identify all patients who will develop complications during the intrapartum period (AAP & ACOG, 1992; Aumann & Baird, 1993). In addition, some patients identified as low-risk by history and physical assessment upon admission also will develop problems or incur adverse outcomes during birth.

Even when antepartal risk scoring is not used, the nurse uses knowledge of maternal-fetal physiology to identify risk factors from the patient's history and current condition. The presence or absence of risk factors helps to identify patients whose condition may warrant more intense maternal or fetal surveillance. Knowledge of specific risk factors in the maternal-fetal history alerts the nurse to potential risks associated with those risk factors. For example, by understanding the physiology of intrauterine growth restriction, the nurse is alert to the possibility of changes in fetal data that may reflect uteroplacental insufficiency. For another example, inadequate nutrition and poor weight gain during the current pregnancy provides information about the potential for placental insufficiency during the antepartum and intrapartum periods. Awareness of the physiologic implications of a risk factor enables the nurse to be alert for a possible adverse response. In addition to these examples of more chronic historical factors, more recent historical data, such as fetal movement status, bleeding, and the status of membranes, must be assessed. Chronic or recent drug ingestion, whether prescriptive or illicit, is another example of a factor that may have an impact on some fetuses. This also has potential implications for fetal well-being, and, therefore, the FHR response.

Obtaining an initial fetal heart assessment also will provide additional information for determining the appropriate method and frequency of subsequent fetal heart assessment.

In summary, maternal-fetal assessment is ongoing and reflects past and current events including the likely effects of labor on fetal well-being.

Maternal-Fetal Physical Assessment

The initial physical assessment of the perinatal patient provides additional data with implications for defining the type and intensity of fetal surveillance needed. Essential elements of initial physical assessment include, but are not limited to

- Abdominal palpation (Leopold's maneuvers) for assessment of fetal position and presentation.
- FHR assessment by fetoscope, Doppler, or electronic fetal monitor.
- Fundal height assessment.
- Maternal vital signs.
- Assessment of edema.
- Urinalysis (dipstick).
- Assessment of vaginal discharge and bleeding.
- Abdominal palpation for uterine resting tone and activity, including assessment of frequency, intensity, and duration of contractions.
- Assessment of labor status by appropriate methods (e.g., cervical examination if no contraindications).

The data from the history and physical assessment often are used to determine the frequency of monitoring needed. Patients who demonstrate greater risk for intrapartum problems can be identified for closer surveillance, while those without current risk or problems can be observed at somewhat longer intervals. For example, the FHR of "high-risk" patients during the active phase of the first stage of labor may be evaluated at 15-minute intervals, whether using auscultation or continuous EFM (ACOG, 1995; AWHONN, 1992). For "low-risk" patients, the FHR may be evaluated at 30-minute intervals during the active phase of labor (ACOG, 1995; AWHONN, 1992). During the second stage of labor, the fetal heart rate is evaluated every 15 minutes for "low risk" patients and every 5 minutes for women with high risk factors (ACOG, 1995; AWHONN, 1992). Similarly, SOGC (1995) has recommended evaluation intervals of every 30 minutes for the latent phase, every 15-30 minutes in the active phase, and every 5 minutes in the second stage of labor.

The nurse also uses the assessment data, together with institutional policy, patient preference, physician or midwife preference, and knowledge of resources available, to determine the type of monitoring to be used. This will be discussed further in the section on techniques. Regardless of the FHM method selected, the physiologic implications of the data base are used to direct the interpretation of and response to subsequent FHR findings.

Physiologic Basis for FHM Interpretation

Accurate FHM assessment is based on understanding the physiology and pathophysiology of fetal heart responses to the intrauterine environment. These responses are indirect indicators of fetal oxygenation. Normal FHR characteristics, including reflex responses to stress, are indicators of adequate oxygenation of the central nervous system (CNS).

The study of maternal and fetal physiology remains an evolving science. Research using animal models, coupled with the ongoing clinical evaluation of associations found between FHR tracings and fetal outcomes, has led to progressive improvement in understanding the process of fetal homeostasis. A relationship among FHR changes, fetal status, fetal oxygenation, and fetal acid-base status exists.

Physiologic controls of the FHR can be divided loosely into FHR influences that are intrinsic to the fetus, those that are extrinsic, and those that represent the homeostatic interaction between the fetus and its environment. Intrinsic factors include the fetal mechanisms of FHR control and related fetal cardiovascular anatomy and physiology. Extrinsic factors include the fetal environment, maternal cardiovascular and uterine anatomy and physiology, and placental and umbilical cord structure and function.

Intrinsic Influences on the FHR

The fetal heart, like the adult heart, has an intrinsic rate which is determined by the dominant pacemaker or sinoatrial (SA) node. The average heart rate range is 110-160 beats per minute (bpm) in the healthy near-term fetus (Parer, 1997).

However, the heart rate in a healthy fetus is rarely static. Normal baseline variations, or variability, as well as more dramatic changes in the rate are present. Several factors interact to influence the rate at which the SA node actually fires. In the healthy fetus, these factors arise primarily from the autonomic nervous system (ANS). Changes also may be related to drugs, cardiac defects in structure or conduction, medications, and levels of oxygen.

The ANS has two branches, sympathetic and parasympathetic, which exert opposing influences on the FHR. Sympathetic stimulation increases FHR, while parasympathetic stimulation decreases FHR. The sympathetic and parasympathetic branches exert their influences in response to information on fetal oxygenation and blood pressure from the chemoreceptors and baroreceptors (Figure 2-2). Chemoreceptors are sensitive to changes in blood O_2, CO_2, and pH levels and are located in the aortic arch, carotid bodies, and medulla oblongata. Baroreceptors are sensitive to changes in blood pressure and are located in the aortic arch and carotid sinuses (Figure 2-2).

The following tables summarize the effects of the ANS, baro- and chemoreceptors, and other intrinsic influences on the FHR.

Parasympathetic nervous system influences

STRUCTURE	FUNCTION
• Vagus nerve, originating in the medulla oblongata. • Innervates the sinoatrial (SA) and the atrioventricular (AV) nodes in the heart.	• Stimulation slows SA node rate of firing, producing a decrease in FHR. • Action occurs via release of acetylcholine. • Tone increases as gestation advances and produces downward effect on baseline rate. • Responsible for producing long-term variability (LTV) and short-term variability (STV) of FHR, with greatest influence on STV. • Effect on FHR may be exaggerated during hypoxemia. • Blocking (e.g., with atropine) produces increased FHR and loss of variability.

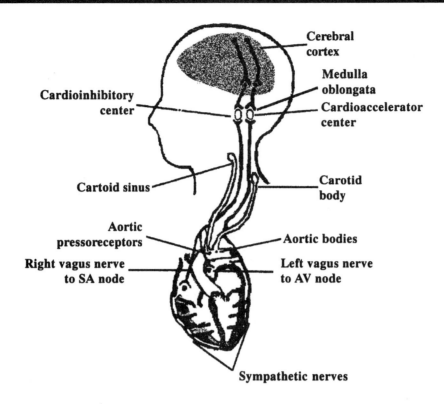

Figure 2-2. Intrinsic influences on the FHR: Baroreceptors, chemoreceptors, autonomic nervous system, and central nervous system.

<u>Sympathetic nervous system influences</u>

<u>STRUCTURE</u>

- Nerves distributed widely in fetal myocardium.

<u>FUNCTION</u>

- Stimulation produces increase in strength of myocardial contraction and increase in FHR.
- Action occurs through release of norepinephrine
- Responsible for long-term baseline variability in conjunction with parasympathetic system.
- Blocking the sympathetic system, as with maternal medication, produces a decrease in the baseline FHR.
- Effect on the FHR may be stimulated during hypoxemia.

Chemoreceptor influences

<table>
<tr><td align="center">STRUCTURE</td><td align="center">FUNCTION</td></tr>
<tr><td>

• Located peripherally (aortic bodies and carotid bodies) and centrally (medulla oblongata).

</td><td>

• Respond to changes in O_2, and CO_2 tensions, and pH levels in blood or cerebrospinal fluid.

• Stimulation due to mild increases in CO_2 or mild decreases in O_2 produces an increase in fetal blood pressure and FHR; more severe changes produce bradycardia.

</td></tr>
</table>

Baroreceptor influences

<table>
<tr><td align="center">STRUCTURE</td><td align="center">FUNCTION</td></tr>
<tr><td>

• Stretch receptors located within vessel walls of the aortic arch and carotid sinus.

• Cardiac responses transmitted via vagus nerve and sympathetic nerves.

</td><td>

• Respond rapidly to changes in fetal blood pressure.

• Increase in fetal blood pressure produces a decrease in the FHR, which decreases fetal cardiac output and blood pressure.

• Decrease in fetal blood pressure results in sympathetic stimulation to increase FHR.

</td></tr>
</table>

Central nervous system influences

<table>
<tr><td align="center">STRUCTURE</td><td align="center">FUNCTION</td></tr>
<tr><td>

• Cerebral cortex.

• Medulla oblongata.

</td><td>

• Responsible for variations in FHR and variability in response to fetal sleep state and body movements.

• Integrative center for central and peripheral neural influences that produces variability and net increase or decrease in baseline FHR.

</td></tr>
</table>

Hormonal influences

HORMONE	FUNCTION
• Catecholamines (Figure 2-3)	• Facilitate hemodynamic changes in response to hypoxemia; facilitate adaptational changes in a neonate at birth (Lagercrantz & Slotkin, 1986; Parer, 1983a, 1989).
• Epinephrine	• Secreted by adrenal medulla (in significantly smaller amounts than norepinephrine).
	• Increases FHR and blood flow to skeletal muscle.
• Norepinephrine (Lagercrantz & Slotkin, 1986; Parer, 1989)	• Predominant hormone secreted by adrenal medulla, also secreted by sympathetic nerves.
	• Associated with initial increase in FHR
	• Increases blood flow to vital organs (brain, heart, adrenals), and away from nonvital organs (e.g., gastrointestinal tract and periphery).
	• The above hemodynamic changes elevate blood pressure and may cause a parasympathetic response that is reflected by a decreased FHR. Norepinephrine cannot overcome this parasympathetic response.
	• Secreted in greater amounts than that found in a resting adult.
• Vasopressin (also known as Arginine Vasopressin Hormone, AVH) (Bissonnette, 1991; Heymann, 1989; Lagercrantz & Slotkin, 1986; Parer, 1989)	• Secreted by pituitary; increased release during hypoxemia and hemorrhage (little influence in unstressed fetus).
	• Helps regulate blood pressure.
	• Produces a rise in blood pressure by increasing peripheral vascular resistance and decreasing FHR.
	• Decreases blood flow to nonvital organs (e.g., gastrointestinal tract and periphery).

- Renin/angiotensin system

  - Renin

    - Secreted by kidneys; increased release in response to hemorrhage (hypovolemia).

  - Angiotensin II (Bissonette, 1991; Heymann, 1989; Lagercrantz & Slotkin, 1986)

    - Secreted by kidneys; increased release in response to hemorrhage and hypoxemia.
    - Exerts tonic vasoconstricting effect on peripheral vascular bed resulting in maintenance of systemic arterial blood pressure and umbilical-placental blood flow.
    - Increased release produces marked increase in blood pressure with an initial decrease in FHR followed by an increase to higher than the previous FHR. Increased release produces increased cardiac output and blood flow to heart.
    - Decreases renal blood flow.

Oxygen Deprivation

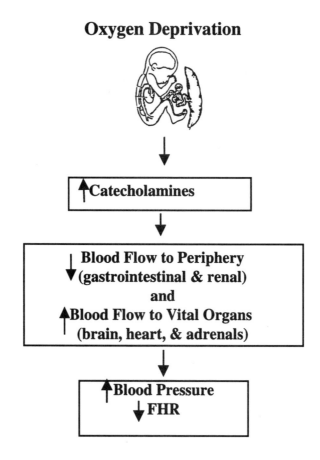

↑Catecholamines

↓ **Blood Flow to Periphery**
↓ **(gastrointestinal & renal)**
and
↑**Blood Flow to Vital Organs**
↑ **(brain, heart, & adrenals)**

↑**Blood Pressure**
↓**FHR**

Increased catecholamine levels cause the peripheral blood flow to decrease while the blood flow to vital organs increases. These flow changes along with the increased catecholamine secretions increase the blood pressure and slow the heart rate.

Figure 2-3. Intrinsic fetal response to oxygen deprivation: Redistribution of blood flow. (Adapted from Lagercrantz & Slotkin, 1986)

Extrinsic Influences on the FHR

Extrinsic influences are the factors in the fetal environment which affect the availability of oxygen and its ability to be transported to the fetus. These factors include maternal factors, uteroplacental factors, umbilical cord factors, and fetal factors which are not part of the intrinsic FHR regulation system.

Maternal Influences

Maternal physiologic influences on the FHR can be viewed in the context of their impact on the availability of oxygen for transport by the placenta and use by the fetus for growth and development. Selected examples of key extrinsic influences are described in the following section.

Baseline maternal arterial oxygen tension is the source for oxygen transported to and used by the fetus.

- Acute maternal hypoxemia compromises maternal arterial oxygen saturation and tension and reduces oxygen available to the fetus.

- Acute or chronic maternal respiratory disease (e.g., acute pulmonary edema, chronic asthma, or cystic fibrosis) may reduce oxygen tension and result in compromised fetal or placental growth and development.

- Maternal smoking results in a lowered oxygen saturation despite adequate oxygenation because carbon monoxide molecules displace oxygen on maternal and fetal hemoglobin.

- Maternal hypoventilation due to breath holding during pushing may transiently decrease oxygen availability.

Maternal oxygen-carrying capacity depends on sufficient hemoglobin to transport oxygen.

- Maternal blood volume increases by approximately 45% during pregnancy due to an increase in plasma volume and an increase in erythrocytes (and, therefore, hemoglobin) of approximately 30%; maternal hematocrit actually decreases due to a dilutional effect.

- Maternal anemia that is due to iron deficiency, hemoglobinopathies (e.g., thalassemia or sickle-cell disease), or hemorrhage reduces available hemoglobin for oxygen transport.

Adequate blood flow to the uterus determines the availability of oxygen for placental perfusion (Figure 2-4).

- Maternal cardiac output increases during pregnancy by approximately 40% in response to the increased volume (size) of the circulatory system. This increased volume is accompanied by peripheral vasodilation and the development of the large vascular bed in the placenta.

- Normal uterine blood flow is determined by adequacy of maternal arterial blood pressure. Supine positioning can significantly reduce uterine blood flow by decreasing venous return and uterine arterial blood pressure. Maternal diseases and drugs that produce significant vasoconstriction reduce uterine blood flow (e.g., hypertensive disorders, vascular disease, and cocaine), likely secondary to increased sympathetic activity or catecholamine production (Kirkinen, Jouppila, Koivula, Vuori, & Puukka, 1983).

- Conduction anesthesia may cause a systemic hypotension, which markedly reduces uterine arterial pressure and, therefore, uterine blood flow.

- Maternal hyperventilation also may increase catecholamine production, exaggerate the mild compensated respiratory alkalemia of pregnancy, and reduce uterine blood flow (maternal hyperventilation may increase the maternal pH to the extent that the fetal pH is elevated even in the presence of fetal acidemia, a potentially confounding factor in the interpretation of fetal scalp sampling data).

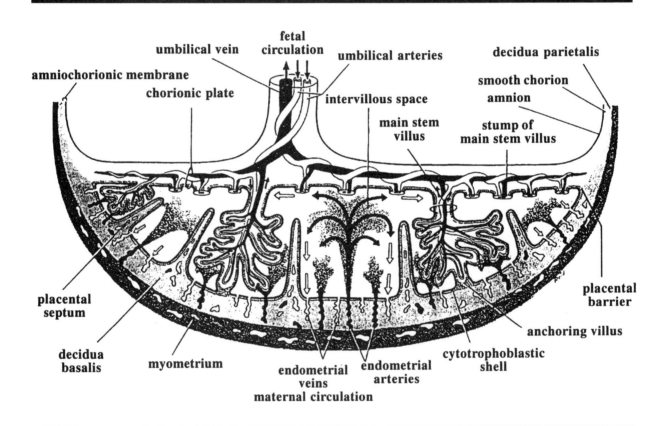

Figure 2-4. As maternal blood enters the intervillous space, it flows upward from uterine spiral arterioles and spreads laterally at random (Moore, 1993).

<u>Uterine contractions</u> influence fetal oxygen availability.

- The myofibrils of the uterus consist of two layers, one circular and one longitudinal. Biochemical and physiologic changes occur near term and during parturition, enabling the uterus to contract in a coordinated, efficient manner. Brief, weak uterine contractions occur early in pregnancy and are replaced by stronger, more regular contractions near term. Progression into labor contractions may be gradual or abrupt (Caldeyro-Barcia & Poseiro, 1960).

- Baseline tonus is a characteristic of the pregnant uterus at rest and represents intrauterine pressure between contractions; pressures greater than 20-25 mm Hg usually are considered hypertonus (Freeman & Garite, 1981).

- Uterine arteries and veins conducting maternal blood to and from the placental circulation pass through the myometrium and are compressed during uterine contractions. During labor, oxygen/carbon dioxide exchange occurs primarily between uterine contractions when blood flow is unimpeded. Uteroplacental blood flow decreases at intrauterine pressures greater than 35 mm Hg and may cease at pressures of approximately 50-60 mm Hg; therefore, some degree of reduction in maternal-fetal exchange will occur during most uterine contractions (Figure 2-5).

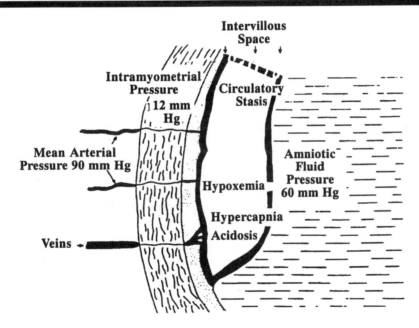

At the acme, or peak of a contraction of greater than 50 mm Hg, uteroplacental blood flow ceases temporarily. This causes the fetus to be dependent upon placental reserve. There may be a brief alteration of contraction effectiveness.

Figure 2-5. Uteroplacental blood flow and the influence of intramyometrial pressure. (Adapted from Freeman, Garite, & Nageotte, 1991; Poseiro, 1969)

<u>Placental Influences</u>

The placental structure and ability to function both affect the availability of oxygen for fetal use, and in turn affect the FHR. Key placental influences include the placental structure, the placental function, and placental blood flow.

<u>Placental Structure</u>

- Functional placental surface area is the amount of placental-fetal interface surface available for the exchange of nutrients (e.g., oxygen, amino acids, proteins, and glucose), elimination of fetal waste, and production of hormones and steroids (Figure 2-6).

- Functional placental surface area depends on adequate maternal nutrients and maternal-uterine blood flow.

<u>Placental Function</u>

- Adequate placental function provides for the transport of oxygen to the fetus at levels above fetal basal needs (e.g., placental reserve) (Meschia, 1985).

- Compromised placental growth and development results in decreased placental function, and may, depending on the degree and timing of compromise, result in fetal growth restriction and, possibly, inadequate oxygenation (Figure 2-7).

- Decreased placental function impairs the fetal ability to withstand the normal stresses of labor and birth (e.g., intrinsic fetal homeostatic mechanisms may be unable to compensate for normal degrees of hypoxemia seen with uterine activity).

- Depending upon the degree of loss of placental function, additional hypoxemic stresses usually tolerated by the healthy fetus may result in rapid decompensation.

- Compromised placental function also may be associated with a reduction of amniotic fluid volume, limiting protection of the fetus and umbilical cord (Clark, 1990; Phelan, 1989).

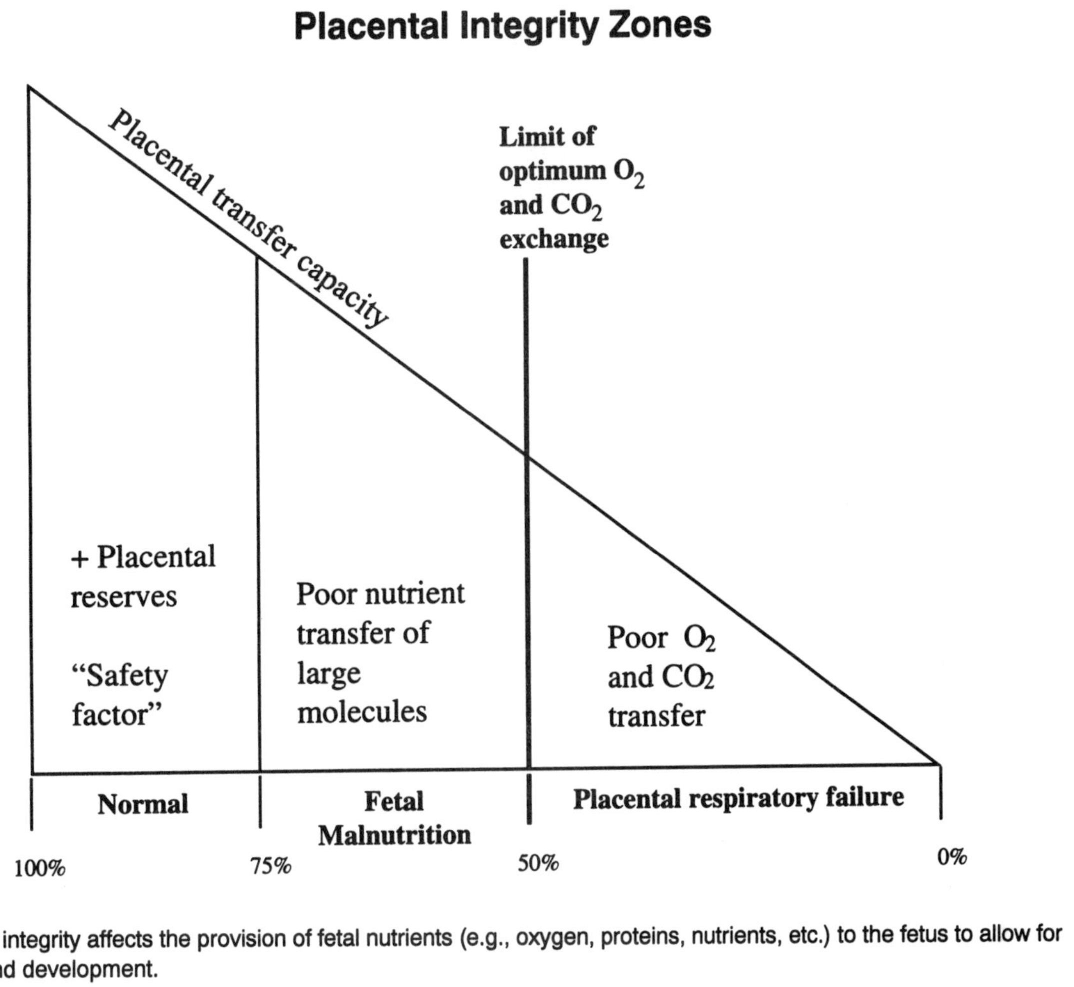

Placental Integrity Zones

Placental transfer capacity

Limit of
optimum O_2
and CO_2
exchange

+ Placental
reserves

"Safety
factor"

Poor nutrient
transfer of
large
molecules

Poor O_2
and CO_2
transfer

Normal   **Fetal
Malnutrition**   **Placental respiratory failure**

100%   75%   50%   0%

Placental integrity affects the provision of fetal nutrients (e.g., oxygen, proteins, nutrients, etc.) to the fetus to allow for growth and development.

Figure 2-6. Placental transfer capacity (Adapted from Parer, 1983b)

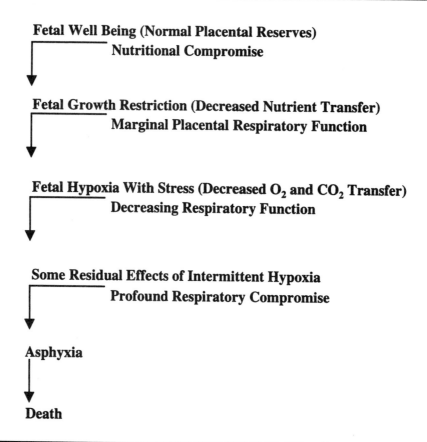

Fetal Well Being (Normal Placental Reserves)
Nutritional Compromise

Fetal Growth Restriction (Decreased Nutrient Transfer)
Marginal Placental Respiratory Function

Fetal Hypoxia With Stress (Decreased O_2 and CO_2 Transfer)
Decreasing Respiratory Function

Some Residual Effects of Intermittent Hypoxia
Profound Respiratory Compromise

Asphyxia

Death

Figure 2-7. Adverse effects of compromised placental functions

Placental blood flow and blood oxygen content affect oxygen delivery to the fetus.

- Approximately 70%-90% of uterine blood flow reaches the placenta. This percentage directly reflects the amount of oxygen available for maternal-fetal exchange (Parer, 1983b).

- Substances cross the placenta by several mechanisms; oxygen is believed to cross the placenta predominantly by simple passive diffusion at a rate directly proportional to placental area and to the differences in concentration and pressures of oxygen on either side.

- Fetal gas exchange occurs in the placental villi contained within the cotyledons (normally 15-30 in number) and depends on the structural integrity of the placenta and the related placental blood flow. Placental structural integrity may be compromised by damage to the cotyledons (infarcts) as seen in maternal conditions such as inadequate nutrition, diabetes, smoking, or preeclampsia.

- Placental aging, partial abruption, and structural abnormalities, such as circumvallate placenta, also may compromise placental integrity, blood flow, and oxygen delivery. These conditions may be observed and evaluated by ultrasound scan.

- Uteroplacental vessels have a marked capacity for constriction in response to either maternal sympathetic nervous system activation or vasoconstrictor drugs. The constricted vessels may result in reduced placental blood flow and reduced fetal gas exchange even in the presence of normal maternal hemoglobin and arterial oxygen saturation (Zuspan, O'Shaughnessy, & Iams, 1981).

Umbilical Cord Influences

The umbilical cord is the vascular connection between the placenta and fetus. The cord's contribution to fetal oxygenation and the subsequent FHR responses may be considered as either extrinsic or intrinsic factors. The umbilical cord has not been shown to have direct innervation. Alterations in blood flow may be attributed to structural, mechanical, or direct fetal myocardial influence (Zuspan, O'Shaughnessy, & Iams, 1981) (Figure 2-8).

- Vascular abnormalities of the cord, such as true knots (Figure 2-9), strictures, or hematomas, may cause an acute or chronic impairment in blood flow.

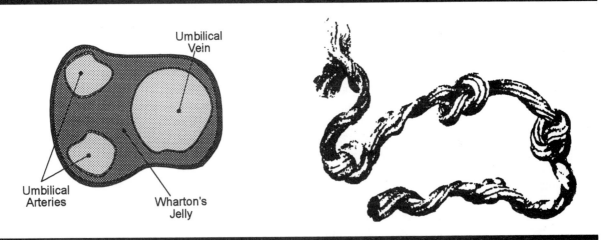

Figure 2-8. Vessels surrounded by Wharton's Jelly, providing protection to umbilical vessels.

Figure 2-9. True knots in the umbilical cord (Maygrier, 1834)

- Impaired blood flow most commonly is due to mechanical forces, such as compression of the umbilical cord by fetal body parts or loops of cord coiled around portions of the fetal body. This type of compression is found intermittently in the majority of labor experiences.
- FHR responses to umbilical cord compression have been shown to vary significantly depending upon the degree of occlusion and the resulting degree of reduction in blood flow (Itskovitz, La Gamma, & Rudolph, 1983).
- In a previously well-oxygenated fetus, partial cord occlusion that results in the occlusion of only the low-pressure umbilical vein may produce a decrease in fetal cardiac output and blood pressure, sympathetic stimulation, and result in an increase in the FHR (James et al., 1976).
- Cord occlusion may produce transient hypoxemia, unless the occlusion is prolonged or chronic.

- Complete, abrupt cord compression results in an abrupt increase in fetal blood pressure that may stimulate fetal baroreceptors and produces an abrupt decrease in FHR; continuation of the complete cord occlusion is likely to result in hypoxemia, chemoreceptor response, and prolongation of decreased FHR. If unrelieved, complete cord compression, as seen with a prolapsed cord, may result in progressive hypoxia and acidosis (James et al., 1976).

Homeostatic Mechanisms

Fetal adaptation to the normal or abnormal stresses of labor and birth occurs through homeostatic mechanisms. These mechanisms provide for reflex responses to hypoxemia and nonhypoxemic stress. The normal healthy fetus is well equipped to withstand the repeated, transient hypoxemia resulting from uterine contractions. However, prolonged or repeated hypoxemia, or a lack of fetal reserves prior to labor, may deplete fetal resources and result in decompensation.

Interpretation of FHR data requires the ability to differentiate among three types of FHR changes: those that result from nonhypoxemic reflex responses, those that result from compensatory responses to hypoxemia, and those that result from impending decompensation. The responses of the fetal heart result from the interplay of intrinsic and extrinsic forces. The fetal physiologic status frequently changes as the fetus responds to the changing environment and the availability of intrinsic resources for homeostasis. This Dynamic Physiologic Response model is illustrated in Figure 2-10.

Several conditions or events have been shown to result in nonhypoxemic reflex responses of the FHR. The respective FHR changes may be the result of direct vagal stimulation, catecholamine release, or baroreceptor response to temporary blood pressure changes in the fetus. Examples of circumstances in which these nonhypoxemic reflex changes in FHR may occur include the following:

- Fetal movement of sufficient intensity and duration may be associated with a temporary increase in FHR secondary to sympathetic nerve stimulation.
- Brief, acute occlusion of the umbilical cord may be associated with a brief increase or decrease in FHR secondary to fetal blood pressure changes alone (prolonged cord occlusion may lead to hypoxemia and chemoreceptor stimulation).
- Head compression occurring at certain periods of labor may be associated with a temporary decrease in the FHR in direct correlation with the intensity and duration of a uterine contraction via vagal stimulation.

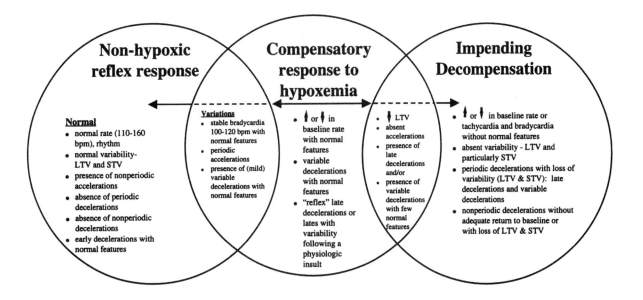

Figure 2-10. Alterations of FHR patterns by dynamic physiologic response

Fetal blood flow channels blood for oxygen delivery via the fetal circulatory system. To enable the oxygenated blood from the placenta to reach the fetal systemic circulation, anatomic vascular shunts are present. These shunts also support preferential blood flow and streaming patterns, which limit the mixing of oxygenated and deoxygenated blood and provide a compensatory response mechanism for decreased umbilical blood flow and hypoxemia (Meschia, 1989). Animal studies demonstrate that circulatory patterns change in response to significant decreases in blood flow by selectively redistributing that blood flow (Meschia, 1989). These circulatory responses are interrelated with autonomic nervous system, chemo- and baroreceptor, and hormonal responses (Figure 2-11).

Intrinsic Fetal Compensation

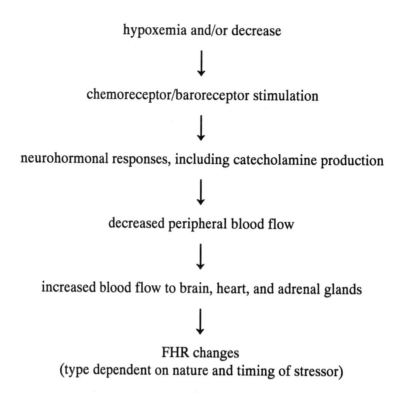

hypoxemia and/or decrease

↓

chemoreceptor/baroreceptor stimulation

↓

neurohormonal responses, including catecholamine production

↓

decreased peripheral blood flow

↓

increased blood flow to brain, heart, and adrenal glands

↓

FHR changes
(type dependent on nature and timing of stressor)

Figure 2-11. Intrinsic fetal compensation (Parer, 1983a)

Fetal Reserve

Fetal reserve is a term representing the concept that the fetus is provided with resources (oxygen and nutrition) in excess of its baseline needs (Parer, 1983a). Specifically, the term refers to the degree of hypoxemia the fetus can tolerate before tissue hypoxia and subsequent acidosis will occur. The following variables in fetal reserve influence the variation in fetal response between individuals:

- Approximately twice as much oxygen is provided to the fetus as would be required normally in the healthy maternal-fetal unit. The amount of oxygen available to the fetus is decreased in situations of intrinsic uteroplacental insufficiency (e.g., in intrauterine growth restriction).

- Oxygen perfusion of fetal organs is greater than normally required by the fetus.

- Preferential blood flow to vital fetal organs can compensate for diminishing reserve capability, but only as long as there is sufficient oxygen to allow the ANS and other compensatory mechanisms (e.g., the adrenal gland) to function normally.

The primary objective of a compensatory response to hypoxemia is maintenance of circulation to the fetal brain (brain-sparing) and the heart to ensure the integrity of cardiac function. Acute hypoxemia in the previously normoxic fetus may produce sympathetic stimulation and acceleration in the FHR (e.g., with acute venous compression in the umbilical cord). Acute hypoxemia also may produce vagal stimulation, with an abrupt decrease in FHR, and decreased oxygen delivery. Baroreceptors, chemoreceptors, and hormonal responses may be involved. Chronic hypoxemia causes prolonged use of physiologic mechanisms and biochemical resources that may result in an inability to compensate when acute hypoxemic events occur. FHR patterns preceding death in the chronically hypoxemic fetus cannot be defined specifically, but all have demonstrated a loss of STV. However, a fetus also may demonstrate the loss of STV without being hypoxemic (e.g., certain dysrhythmias).

The ongoing observation of the fetal heart response as a major determinant of fetal status during the antepartum and intrapartum period reflects the likelihood of specific physiologic mechanisms, reserves, and conditions. Measurement of the FHR and its response to uterine activity can be accomplished by several methods. Selection of the method to evaluate these fetal heart changes and uterine activity is determined by various factors discussed in the next section.

Techniques of Fetal Heart Monitoring

The primary purpose of FHM is to obtain data on the FHR response to make appropriate diagnostic and management decisions. For several decades, continuous electronic FHM has been used widely for fetal assessment during labor and birth. This technology has been adopted for use with both low- and high-risk patients. Some experts have recommended the use of auscultation for low-risk patients during labor as the primary monitoring technique (SOGC, 1995).

Clearly, a lack of consensus exists regarding the actual effectiveness of electronic FHM in comparison with traditional techniques of auscultation. Some clinicians question the necessity of incorporating technology into every labor and birth experience (Snydal, 1988; Supplee & Vezeau, 1996). Others maintain that the use of electronic FHM unnecessarily increases the cesarean rate with no demonstrable improvements in neonatal outcomes (McCusker, Harris, & Hosmer, 1988). Although randomized, prospective clinical trials of EFM have been published, there is not universal agreement on the conclusions that may be drawn from those studies (Thacker, Stroup, & Peterson, 1995; Vintzileos et al., 1995; Vintzileos et al., 1993). The results of research on the risks and benefits of electronic FHM, while still controversial, have led to recent alterations in published guidelines of practice for FHR assessment during labor (ACOG, 1995, 1989a; SOGC, 1995). The revised guidelines do not stipulate that any particular type of patient is required to be monitored by EFM. Instead, guidelines for auscultation and EFM of both low and high-risk patients are described.

Ultimately, the selection of an FHM method rests on a combination of factors. In some settings, institutional policies and procedures dictate a specific methodology. In other settings, selection is determined by clinician or patient preference. Other institutions and individuals may discriminate between risk groups, allowing auscultation alone only for those patients in whom risk factors are absent. The selection and appropriate use of FHM techniques relies on a thorough nursing assessment and diagnosis of the individual patient's needs.

In some clinical environments, the lack of sufficient numbers of nurses with appropriate expertise in auscultatory techniques has limited the use of auscultation as an alternative to electronic FHM. In addition, the time available for auscultation to meet a 1:1 nurse-to-fetus ratio is sometimes limited (Morrison et al., 1993). In other clinical environments, legal risks and a preference to access FHR data have resulted in the continuing use of electronic FHM.

Appropriate FHR assessment considers both electronic and nonelectronic techniques for acquiring the FHR and uterine activity data. Regardless of the FHM method selected for a given patient, the nurse is accountable for knowing how to recognize and respond to auditory, as well as electronically obtained, FHR data. FHR data must be simultaneously assessed with uterine activity. The nurse also must know how to recognize and respond to both palpated and electronically obtained uterine activity data.

Developing skills in both methods enables the nurse to select and combine techniques as needed to provide optimal care for individual patients, and allows the nurse to respond to patient, care provider, and institutional preferences. The following section describes and discusses various methods of monitoring, beginning with the nonelectronic methods of auscultation and palpation; progressing to the electronic detection of uterine activity via the tocodynamometer, fluid-filled intrauterine pressure catheter (IUPC) and sensor-tipped or solid-state IUPC; and ending with electronic detection of the FHR via ultrasound and spiral electrode placement.

Nonelectronic Techniques of Monitoring

Auscultation and Palpation Assessment

Auscultation of the fetal heart and abdominal palpation of uterine activity have been important dimensions of obstetric care for several centuries and remain key assessments. There has been a recent renewed interest in using intermittent auscultation as a primary fetal assessment method. A brief discussion of some issues surrounding the use of intermittent auscultation will be presented prior to reviewing the capabilities, limitations, and techniques of auscultation and palpation.

Auscultation

As stated in a previous section, research on the effectiveness and efficacy of intermittent auscultation versus EFM has been done over the past 20 to 30 years. Researchers in randomized controlled trials have not demonstrated clear, consistent differences in neonatal outcomes between intermittent auscultation and continuous EFM groups. Although one recent randomized clinical trial indicated a significant decrease in perinatal death in the EFM group (Vintzileos et al., 1993), meta-analyses of multiple randomized trials have not demonstrated consistent differences in neonatal deaths (Thacker, Stroup, & Peterson, 1995; Vintzileos et al., 1995). A reduction of neonatal seizures was found in one

40

study (Thacker et al., 1995), although the seizures did not persist over time. On the basis of randomized clinical trial findings to date, the equivalence of intermittent auscultation and EFM has been assumed (ACOG, 1995; SOGC, 1995). However, the issue of standardization of terminology, interpretation, and management of fetal heart patterns has not been consistently addressed between studies. This has been recognized and will be addressed in future research (Bernardes, 1996; Parer, 1996; Thacker & Stroup, 1996).

Additional research also may provide further information about who needs to be monitored with which method, when, and for how long. Research clarifying the capabilities and limitations of both methods of monitoring will be useful in guiding practice. For example, auscultation in nonstress testing has been used effectively to detect accelerations when compared with EFM (Paine, 1992). In contrast, continuous EFM during labor was more likely to result in detection of all types of acidemia at birth than intermittent auscultation based on a re-analysis of data from a randomized trial comparing intermittent auscultation and continuous EFM (Vintzileos et al., 1995). Although there was not a significant difference of the rate of acidemia between groups, in the EFM group, nonreassuring FHR patterns were identified in 21 of 22 fetuses with metabolic acidosis, 20 of 21 fetuses with mixed acidosis, and 23 of 23 fetuses with respiratory acidosis. In the intermittent auscultation group, nonreassuring FHR patterns were identified in 5 of 19 fetuses with metabolic acidosis, 6 of 16 fetuses with mixed acidosis, and 5 of 12 fetuses with respiratory acidosis. It is interesting to note that intermittent auscultation was done according to ACOG guidelines using a Doppler ultrasound device at least every 15 minutes during the active stage of labor and every 5 minutes in the second stage in this study. Auscultation may be more useful in detecting accelerations as a reassuring finding. In the absence of accelerations, additional information from an EFM method may be needed to provide reassurance of baseline variability that cannot be obtained with auscultation.

An additional issue is the need for adequate resources to be allocated for education of nurses and care providers performing auscultation (Morrison et al., 1993). Auscultation requires different skills, including auditory recognition of changes in the FHR and practical experience in the techniques of auscultation. The need for these resources has been recognized by some professionals advocating the use of intermittent auscultation as a primary method of fetal surveillance in labor (SOGC, 1995).

The issue of adequate resources to ensure a one-to-one nurse-to-fetus ratio is addressed when using auscultation as a primary method of surveillance (NAACOG, 1990; ACOG, 1995; SOGC, 1995; Morrison et al., 1993). A skilled obstetric nurse was in constant attendance during labor and performed auscultation of the FHR every 15 minutes during active labor and every 5 minutes during the second stage in the randomized clinical trials used to support equivalence of auscultation and EFM. Clinical trials comparing different time frames for assessment have not been done.

In addition, true auscultation has been historically associated with using a device, such as a fetoscope, that allows for listening to the actual heart sounds. Currently, the word auscultation is used to imply use of a stethoscope device or a hand-held Doppler ultrasound device (ACOG, 1995; SOGC, 1995, NAACOG, 1990). It is important to keep in mind the capabilities and limitations of the particular device being used when auscultating. For example, a fetoscope is used to detect the auditory signal of the opening and closing of heart values, while a doptone (ultrasound) detects the cardiac motion versus actual heart sounds.

In summary, future research in these areas will continue to emerge and further clarify who needs to be monitored, with what method, when, and how often. With the current focus in health care on promoting consumer satisfaction and quality clinical outcomes in a cost-effective manner, further research will be needed to address these issues. The cost issues associated with the implementation of auscultation and EFM need to be considered, including education of staff and provision of adequate numbers of staff to perform auscultation. Regardless of which method of fetal surveillance is used, auscultation or EFM, a clear understanding of the underlying physiology and the capabilities and limitations of the methods is required.

Auscultation Capabilities

When auscultation is used, the practitioner's assessment is the sole source of information about the FHR. Careful listening and precise descriptions of auscultation findings can provide useful information regarding the fetal status as listed below.

Auscultation detects:

- FHR baseline.
- FHR rhythm.
- Increases and decreases of the FHR.
- Differentiation of the fetal and maternal heart rates, eliminating errors that are due to misplacement of a monitor device or fetal demise.
- Verification of fetal heart dysrhythmias visualized on EFM tracing (fetoscope only).
- Clarification of halving or doubling on the EFM tracing.

Auscultation Limitations

Limitations exist with the auscultation method despite careful listening and descriptions of the FHR by practitioners. A list of some limitations follows.

Auscultation:
- Does not detect LTV or STV.
- Is not continuous and may, therefore, miss or delay detection of decreases and increases of the FHR.

42

- Does not generate a graphic record for assistance in decision-making or future review.
- Requires education, practice, skill, and a 1:1 nurse:fetus ratio.
- May be disrupted by uterine contractions.
- May be limited by position and movement of the mother or fetus, as well as maternal size.

Auscultation Techniques

Auscultation requires use of a fetoscope or pinard stethoscope (type of device) for the assessment of heart sounds. In practice, however, the term auscultation often is used to refer to the assessment of fetal heart sounds by means of a hand-held Doppler device or the ultrasound monitor (ACOG, 1995; SOGC, 1995). Little significant difference exists between the two methods of auscultation except in selected circumstances. For example, when the possibility of a fetal dysrhythmia exists, use of a nonelectronic device will validate heart sounds and rhythms versus the heart motion detected by ultrasound devices. The hand-held Doppler device functions in a similar manner as the Doppler used in electronic fetal monitors except that no permanent recording is produced. Factors to consider when using the hand-held Doppler are listed below.

- Doppler converts movement into sound and amplifies it.
- Improper placement of the device may result in artifact due to displacement of a sonic beam (e.g, detection of maternal heart rate versus FHR).
- Fetal or maternal movement also may result in artifact or counting of reflections from moving fetal-maternal structures.
- Maternal heart rate must be verified (as with other FHM methods) to avoid mistaking the mother's heartbeat for the FHR.
- Assessing the FHR with a Doppler device during a contraction may be easier and more comfortable for the patient

Regardless of the device used in auscultation, skill in sound differentiation is required. The regular rhythm of the FHR must be distinguished from the somewhat similar sounds produced by the maternal vessels (uterine bruit or uterine souffle), sounds that are synchronous with the maternal pulse. Either sound may present clinical problems if confused with the FHR, due to erroneous conclusions regarding fetal status. An elevated maternal heart rate could be mistaken for a normal FHR and result in failure to assess the fetus at all. The passage of blood through the umbilical arteries also produces a double sound (funic souffle). The sound usually has a "swooshing" or "hissing" quality, similar to the heart sounds. Routine assessment of the maternal pulse simultaneous with FHR auscultation is the primary approach to avoid confusion.

Although there are generally accepted techniques for FHR auscultation, these will vary somewhat in individual cases according to the nature of the FHR data sought and clinical circumstances.

Procedure

The recommended procedure for FHR auscultation includes: palpation of the maternal abdomen to locate the fetal back to place the auscultation device; palpation of the maternal pulse to differentiate the FHR; palpation of the uterus to determine the presence of contractions; and counting after and between uterine contractions to identify the baseline FHR, rhythm and responses to contractions (Table 2-1). If possible, counting also is done during contractions. The presence or absence of FHR changes from the baseline may be detected best by auscultation both during and immediately following uterine contractions. Because both types of FHR data are pertinent to providing care, listening at a combination of times is necessary to obtain maximal information. Recommendations include auscultating during a uterine contraction, if possible, and for the 30 second interval following a uterine contraction (NAACOG, 1990). Auscultating for longer periods (60 seconds) after uterine contractions also has been recommended (SOGC, 1995).

Counting for multiple, consecutive periods may help the practitioner in identifying the baseline rate and changes from the baseline. For example, the practitioner may count for consecutive intervals of 6 seconds. The duration of the auscultation period can vary from these multiple brief periods to longer periods (30-60 seconds). Under some circumstances, many practitioners prefer to listen for several continuous minutes.

Frequency of Assessment

The frequency of auscultation assessment and documentation has been a subject of debate. Recommendations for the frequency of auscultation during the latent or early phases of labor vary from intervals of 15, 30, and 60 minutes to not at all (Bobak, Jensen, & Zalar, 1989; Olds, London, & Ladewig, 1992; Snydal, 1992). FHR assessment is a dimension of ongoing labor evaluation. FHR assessment also is required for women being observed for possible labor prior to formal hospital admission. When auscultation is used as the primary FHR monitoring technique in these circumstances, a policy describing the frequency of FHR assessment during the observation period is recommended. In view of the practical realities of risk management principles alone, the patient in possible labor or the latent phase should have the FHR assessed at least as often as the maternal vital signs. The institutional protocol for frequency of FHR auscultation should be based upon facility and practitioner experience as well as recommendations provided by respected professionals (ACOG, 1995; NAACOG, 1990; SOGC, 1995) (Table 2-2).

The recommended frequency of intermittent auscultation during the active phase of labor has ranged from every 15 to 30 minutes depending on risk status (ACOG, 1995; NAACOG, 1990; SOGC, 1995). There is no research to indicate an optimal frequency in absence of risk factors (ACOG, 1995). It has been suggested that in the absence of risk factors, auscultation after a uterine contraction every 30 minutes during the active phase of labor and every 15 minutes during the second stage of labor may be appropriate (ACOG, 1995; NAACOG, 1990; AWHONN, 1992). In the presence of risk factors, auscultation should occur at 15-minute intervals during the active phase and every 5 minutes during the second stage of labor (ACOG, 1995; NAACOG, 1990; AWHONN, 1992). The SOGC has recommended auscultation every 30 minutes during the latent phase, every 15 to 30 minutes during the active phase, and every 5 minutes in the second stage when pushing begins for all patients (SOGC, 1995).

Recommended Procedure for FHR Auscultation

- Palpate the maternal abdomen to identify fetal presentation and position (Leopold's maneuvers).

- Place the bell of the fetoscope or Doppler over the area of anticipated maximum intensity of fetal heart sounds (usually over the fetal back).

- Palpate the maternal radial pulse to differentiate maternal heart rate from FHR.

- Palpate uterine contractions during auscultation to clarify the relationship between FHR and uterine contractions.

- Count the FHR during a uterine contraction if possible, and for at least 30 to 60 seconds thereafter to identify fetal response (NAACOG, 1990).

- Count the FHR between uterine contractions for at least 30 to 60 seconds to identify an average baseline rate (ACOG, 1995; NAACOG, 1990; SOGC, 1995).

- If distinct differences are noted between counts, recount for longer periods to clarify the presence and nature of FHR changes.

- In clarifying accelerations, count for multiple, consecutive, brief periods of 6 seconds and multiply by 10 to establish rate changes.

Table 2-1. Recommended Procedure for FHR Auscultation (ACOG, NAACOG, 1990; SOGC, 1995)

Frequency of Auscultation: Assessment and Documentation

	LATENT	ACTIVE	SECOND STAGE
ACOG			
Low Risk	—	q 30 min	q 15 min
High Risk	—	q 15 min	q 5 min
AWHONN/NAACOG			
Low Risk	q 1 hour	q 30 min	q 15 min
High Risk	q 30 min	q 15 min	q 5 min
SOGC			
All	q 30 min	q 15-30 min	q 5 min

Labor Events

Assess and document FHR prior to
- initiation of labor-enhancing procedures (e.g., artificial rupture of membranes).
- ambulation.
- administration of medications.
- administration of analgesia/anesthesia.

Assess and document FHR following
- rupture of membranes.
- recognition of abnormal uterine activity patterns.
- evaluation of oxytocin (maintenance, increase, or decrease of the dosage).
- administration of medications (at time of peak action) also during and following placement of epidural.
- expulsion of enema.
- catheterization.
- vaginal examination.
- ambulation.
- evaluation of analgesia and/or anesthesia (maintenance, increase, or decrease the dosage).

Table 2-2. Frequency of auscultation: Assessment and documentation (ACOG, 1995; SOGC, 1995; AWHONN, 1992; NAACOG, 1990).

Abdominal Palpation

Uterine activity assessment includes the identification of contraction characteristics, evaluation of uterine resting tone (tonus), and observing for possible abnormal contraction or labor patterns (Table 2-2). Abdominal palpation remains a basic skill of perinatal maternal-fetal assessment regardless of the FHM technique selected for labor surveillance. Abdominal palpation using Leopold's maneuvers is a standard method of assessing fetal position and presentation. In relation to FHM, these four maneuvers provide a systematic approach to identifying the point of maximal sound intensity of the FHR (Figure 2-13). Once this point is identified, the auscultation device or the Doppler ultrasound transducer can be placed in the optimal position for fetal heart assessment.

FHR AUSCULTATION
Interpretation and Intervention/Management

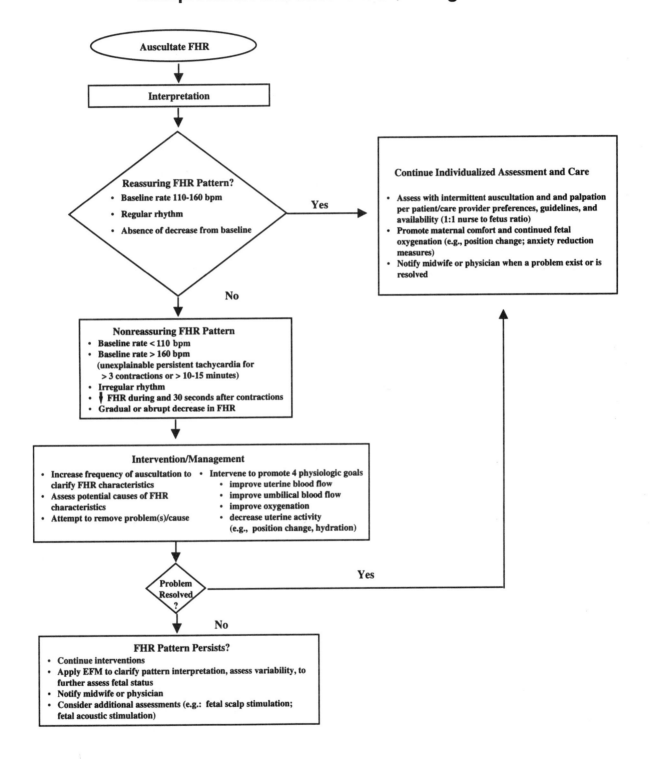

Figure 2-12. FHR auscultation: Interpretation and intervention/management

Leopold's Maneuvers

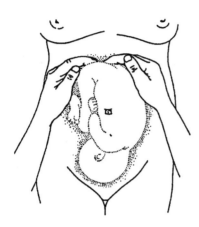

1st Maneuver
Assess part of fetus
in the upper uterus

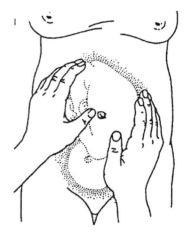

2nd Maneuver
Assess location
of the fetal back

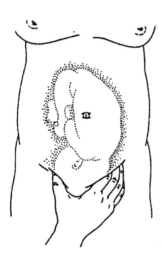

3rd Maneuver
Identify presenting part

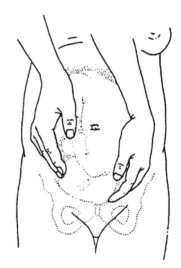

4th Maneuver
Determine the descent
of the presenting part

Figure 2-13. The four steps in performing Leopold's maneuvers (Adapted from Oxorn, 1986; Simpson & Creehan, 1996)

Palpation is best performed by placing the fingers over the fundal area to feel the uterus rise upward as the contraction develops. The sensitive fingertips, rather than the palm surface of the hands, are placed firmly, but without excessive pressure or movement, on the uterus.

Although no standard definition exists for palpated measurement of contraction intensity, many nurses use the following comparison model in the clinical setting (Table 2-3).

The method of describing palpation is based on the degree of indentation that can be introduced in the uterine muscle. If no indentation is possible during a contraction, the contraction is usually described as normal or strong. If the fingertips are able to indent the uterine muscle, the contraction usually is described as subnormal or mild. Describing contractions as "good" is inappropriate. The true effectiveness of contractions can be evaluated only retrospectively (e.g., after a normal labor and delivery process).

Analogy of Contraction Intensity Using Palpation

Contraction Intensity	Corresponds to Palpation of Body Part
mild	tip of nose
moderate	chin
strong	forehead

Table 2-3. Analogy of Contraction Intensity Using Palpation (Malinowski, Pedigo, & Phillips, 1989)

Electronic Techniques of Monitoring

EFM remains an evolving science from both the physiologic and technologic perspectives. The continuous monitoring of both uterine activity and FHR may be recorded by using an external or an internal mode, sometimes referred to as indirect and direct methods. In the United States and Canada, the recommended paper speed of the electronic fetal monitor is 3 cm per minute (ACOG, 1995; SOGC, 1995). Awareness of this is especially important when evaluating tracings from another country or when viewing a tracing that looks especially compact, narrow, or unusual.

Uterine Assessment

Tocodynamometer

Tocotransducers or tocodynamometers are used externally to detect change in the configuration of the uterus as it contracts and hardens. The uterus rises as the intensity of the uterine contraction increases, causing the maternal abdominal wall to rise, and this is detected by a pressure sensor placed on the abdominal wall. Pressure from the uterus causes a spring or button on the sensor to move and that mechanical motion is converted to an electrical signal. These instruments use computer chip technology to sense pressure changes.

Benefits
- Is noninvasive.
- Provides information on uterine relative contraction frequency, duration, and configuration.
- Can be used antepartum and intrapartum with intact or ruptured membranes.
- May be more sensitive to the onset and duration (not intensity) of uterine contractions than the palpating hand of many clinicians, especially if the patient is obese or restless.

Limitations
- Unable to detect uterine contraction intensity and resting tone.
- Unable to accurately detect exact frequency and duration in some cases, such as obesity and preterm labor.
- Is location-sensitive, placement can lead to false information; should be placed where maximum change occurs, a site best located by palpation (Figure 2-14).
- Sensitive to maternal and fetal motion that may be superimposed on waveform (Figure 2-14).

When a tocodynameter is used, palpation of the uterus is used to verify contraction frequency and duration and to assess relative intensity and resting tone. Additionally, asking the mother's perception of her uterine contractions is also useful in evaluating the data generated by the tocodynamometer.

Tocodynamometer Variations

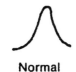
Normal

1. Uterine contraction wave form.

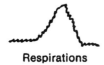
Respirations

2. Respiration may produce an undulating overlay.

Pushing

3. Valsalva maneuver with pushing effects during the second stage of labor may produce blunted spikes.

Vomiting seizures

4. Extreme maternal activity such as vomiting or a seizure may produce a series of sharp spikes.

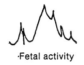
·Fetal activity

5. Fetal movement may produce sharp isolated spikes.

Sudden baseline shift

6. Sudden baseline shifts may be produced by maternal position change.

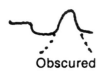
Obscured

7. Low baseline setting may obscure all but tip of contractions.

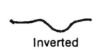
Inverted

8. Certain placements of tocodynamometer may produce reversed waveform when uterus contracts away from the tocodynamometer

Figure 2-14. Tocodynamometer variations (Adapted from Wagner and Cabaniss, unpublished)

Intrauterine Pressure Assessment

Intrauterine pressure catheters (IUPC) are inserted internally to measure the pressures and characteristics of uterine activity: resting tone and contraction, intensity, frequency, and duration. The decision to use an IUPC is based on the clinical need for additional information, to perform amnioinfusion, physician or CNM preference, institutional policy, and availability. There are several types of IUPCs. Key concepts related to fluid-filled and solid sensor-tipped IUPCs are highlighted below.

Fluid-Filled Catheter

A sterile, flexible catheter inserted into the uterus through a guide can be used after rupture of the membranes to monitor the intrauterine pressure directly. The proximal end of the catheter is attached to a pressure transducer. The catheter will measure pressure within the uterine cavity by fluid being displaced with increased pressure. This displaced fluid exerts pressure on the transducer. Pressure against a diaphragm with the transducer generates changes in the electrical resistance of a series of wires. These electrical changes are converted to changes in pressure as measured in millimeters of mercury and displayed on the uterine activity channel of the chart record. This method requires calibration (zeroing) to room air (atmospheric pressure) to remain sensitive to the changes in uterine tonus. The gauge is set at zero by opening the system to air using a three-way stopcock placed at a level midway between the maternal back and the uterine fundus while supine.

The fluid-filled IUPC system is based on the assumption that the intrauterine and intracatheter fluid forms a closed system. The intrauterine pressure generated by a contraction will be transmitted up the fluid column directly to the pressure transducer. This is explained by Pascal's law, which states that the pressure within a fluid-filled closed spheroid is equal at all points.

The accuracy of this system, therefore, depends on the adequacy of the fluid pool surrounding the catheter tip. Intrauterine pressures have been shown to vary by as much as 25% when measured at different areas of the uterus. Other factors also may influence the accuracy of measured pressures. Air in the closed system will cushion the pressure generated, producing a dampened waveform. Leakage and obstruction of the catheter also will distort the wave form (Hutson & Petrie, 1986; Klapholz, 1978).

The self-test button on the fetal monitor is used to verify the proper functioning of the internal circuitry of the equipment. However, this self-test does not ensure that the equipment is properly calibrated. Improper calibration can be a major source of technical error affecting the uterine activity print out. Users of fluid-filled transducers will find detailed instructions for calibration in the operators' manuals supplied by the transducer manufacturers. When calibration has been verified, the catheter can then be accurately zeroed and used.

Benefits

- An accurate method of assessing uterine pressure during contractions and at rest; measured in mm Hg (millimeters of mercury).
- More accurate timing of FHR changes with uterine activity.
- Aspiration of amniotic fluid to assess for chorioamnionitis or fetal lung maturity can be performed.
- Amnioinfusion can be performed.

Limitations

- Rupture of membranes and adequate cervical dilatation are required.
- Procedure is invasive.
- Risk of infection and uterine perforation is increased.
- Careful attention to technique is required, especially when zeroing and calibrating to obtain accurate data.
- Catheter tip may become wedged against fetal part and prevent the production of any pressure data or produce a distorted, damped, or truncated pressure wave.
- Catheter tip position in relation to external pressure transducer position may affect pressures.
- Catheter may become obstructed by particulate matter such as meconium or blood.
- Use may be contraindicated with certain infections where rupture of membranes is discouraged to prevent maternal-to-fetal transmission (e.g., herpes, HIV).
- Pressure readings may be lower than sensor-tipped (or solid) catheter.

Solid Pressure Catheter

An alternative system for monitoring intrauterine pressure was introduced during the last decade (Strong & Paul, 1989). This new technology uses a solid-state micropressure transducer located at the catheter tip. Dual lumen versions that enable simultaneous amnioinfusion or sampling of amniotic fluid and rezeroing after insertion also are available.

Benefits

- Can be zeroed to atmospheric pressure easily. Additionally, most models may be rezeroed as needed during monitoring.
- Design avoids pressure artifacts that may be caused by a catheter containing air or becoming kinked.
- As with fluid-filled catheters, this method provides an accurate assessment of uterine activity, in particular, intensity and resting tone pressures.
- Most models allow amnioinfusion and aspiration of amniotic fluid (see fluid-filled catheter benefits).

Limitations

- Rigidity of catheter tip in some models requires greater degree of caution in placement to avoid possible uterine, placental, or cord perforation.
- Maternal position change may change hydrostatic pressure within the uterus and may alter readings, including data regarding uterine resting tone. Proper use requires baseline readings in the left, right, and supine with lateral tilt positions (Figure 2-15).
- Pressure readings may be higher than with fluid-filled catheters.
- The same limitations of fluid-filled catheters also pertain to sensor-tipped catheters.

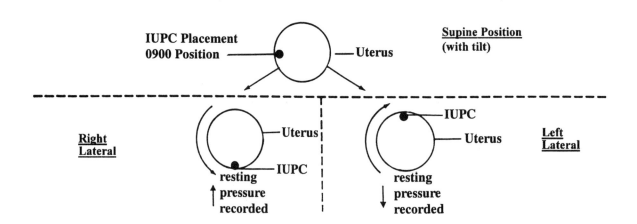

Baseline Readings of Sensor-tipped IUPC After Insertion

Intrauterine hydrostatic pressure is altered by changes in maternal position. Obtaining baseline pressure readings in the left, right, and supine with lateral tilt positions demonstrates these alterations and prevents potential misinterpretation of values following subsequent position changes during labor. The position of the catheter in relation to position of the patient may affect the amount of pressure exerted by the fluid above the catheter. Note that in this position, the right-sided position, the fluid above the catheter is increased (increased internal hydrostatic pressure), thereby adding to or increasing the baseline resting tone. Knowing these baseline differences will prevent erroneous conclusions regarding management of induction or augmentation. This technique is especially helpful when using a single lumen catheter which cannot be rezeroed after it is placed in the patient.

Figure 2-15. Baseline readings of sensor-tipped IUPC after insertion (Adapted from Utah Medical)

Indications for Intrauterine Pressure Monitoring

The fluid-filled and sensor-tipped intrauterine pressure catheters may be used to measure uterine activity in cases of :

- Labor dystocia.

- Previous uterine scar.

- The patient undergoing oxytocin induction and augmentation when external methods of assessing uterine activity are inadequate.

- Amnioinfusion.

Various methods or combinations of methods may be used to assess uterine activity. The decision of whether to use an external or internal method of monitoring will depend on the individual situation. The type of method used will determine the type of information obtained about uterine activity (Figure 2-16). Palpation of uterine activity remains important regardless of the EFM method chosen to confirm uterine activity, uterine resting tone, and/or functioning of the equipment.

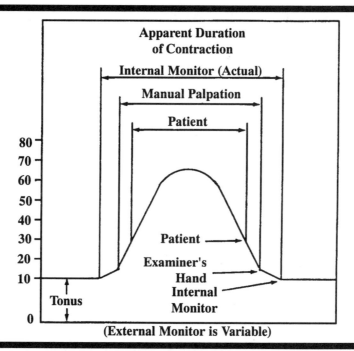

Figure 2-16. Comparison of uterine contraction assessment by palpation, external tocodynamometer, and intrauterine pressure catheter (Freeman et al., 1991)

Fetal Heart Assessment

Ultrasound

The ultrasound device used by the electronic fetal monitor is a Doppler ultrasound transducer. Fetal monitors use a transducer with multiple piezoelectric crystals. These crystals, under electrical stimulation, generate ultrasound waves and receive the reflected ultrasound waves. The waves returning from moving structures are altered in frequency from those of the originally transmitted sound waves. This frequency shift, called the Doppler Shift, is detected and amplified to produce an ultrasound waveform which is interpreted by the computer in the fetal monitor. The monitor processes the waveforms, adds an audible sound, and records the detected FHR. Currently, two methods can be used to analyze fetal cardiac waveforms obtained by ultrasound. These methods are commonly referred to as first and second generation or first generation and autocorrelation. With both methods, the waveforms are detected by a piezoelectric effect (Figure 2-17).

Benefits

- Noninvasive.

- Membranes need not be ruptured.

- Relatively consistent recordings if placed correctly.

- FHR recorded for assessment and permanent record.

- Less personnel-intensive than auscultation.

Limitations

- Restricts patient movement.

- Measures cardiac motion (versus heart sounds) and cannot be used to differentiate dysrhythmias.

- Ultrasound reflections may be weak or absent, and false FHR patterns may be produced when the fetus gradually moves out of the field.

- Episodic maternal and fetal movement may interfere with recording.

- Half counting of FHR may occur, especially in the presence of FHR tachycardia greater than 240 bpm.

- Double counting of the FHR may occur with first generation monitors, although less likely with 2nd generation monitors. MHR may be doubled with either 1st or 2nd generation monitors.

- Artifact may affect the appearance of variability (e.g., may appear as present when actually decreased or absent).

Piezoelectric Effect

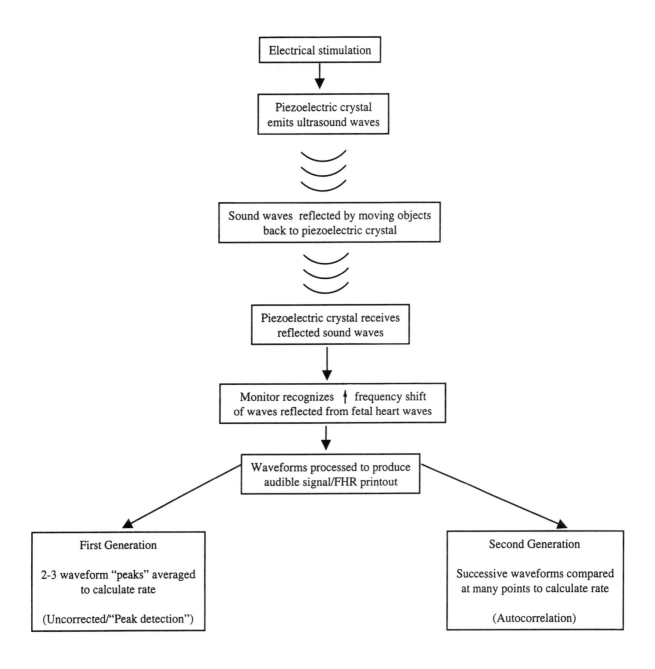

This is a linear view, but in fact, the piezoelectric crystal is emitting and receiving sound waves continually.

Figure 2-17. Linear pictorial of piezoelectric effect (Hon, 1975; Klavan, Laver, & Boscola, 1977)

The electronic system calculates the FHR based on Doppler-generated waveforms. Two issues may affect accuracy when calculating the FHR. First, the electronic fetal monitor must accurately distinguish the fetal cardiac waveform from those generated by fetal chest or limb movements and numerous other artifactual echoes. The monitor also must count the fetal cardiac waveforms accurately. Second, the typical fetal waveform is complex and variable, with one major component generated by the fetal heart valve's motion during systole and the other during diastole. Fetal or maternal movement may cause amplitude changes, fading of signal, and variations in the maximum peaks of these waveforms.

First Generation Monitors

In the evolution of the technology of Doppler FHR assessment, advances in the electronic processing of data have led to a discrimination between two generations of equipment (Boehm et al., 1986). To compensate for the complexity and variation in waveforms, the first-generation monitors employ two mechanisms: use of a refractory window and maximum peak detection.

To prevent the counting of both components of the fetal cardiac waveform as separate beats, a refractory window is used (Hutson & Petrie, 1986; Klapholz, 1978). This window is an inhibitory period during which time the system does not attempt to count the incoming signal. This time period follows the moment of detection of the fetal cardiac waveform and is presumed to be the waveform's first component. The length of time, measured in milliseconds, of the refractory window is dynamic in that the time is set to vary according to the FHR. This variance, however, has limitations. Slow FHRs below 90 bpm may cause the second component of the waveform to occur after the refractory window period. This action will produce a double counting of a single waveform leading to doubling on the FHR tracing. Rapid FHRs may cause a second waveform to occur within the refractory window period and produce halving of the FHR tracing because the second heart beat is not counted.

The complexity and variability of the first generation Doppler-generated waveforms make accurate counting of the same point in the fetal cardiac cycle difficult. The mechanism first-generation monitors use to compensate for this problem is maximum peak detection (Figure 2-18). When the movement of the fetal heart generates a waveform, the monitor detects its maximum peak and then counts the time interval between peaks. Problems with this technique are caused by Doppler signals from other anatomy, such as the umbilical cord, as well as variations in an early or late appearance of the peak in the waveform. These problems lead to false variability or jitter in the printed fetal heart tracing. Consequently, the STV on the tracing cannot be equated with the true status of the fetal heart's STV if a first generation monitor is used.

Second Generation Monitors and Autocorrelation

The major alteration in Doppler signal processing associated with second-generation fetal monitors is referred to by one manufacturer as autocorrelation (Hewlett-Packard, 1984). This technique evolved from efforts to improve the quality of the processing of waveforms. The rapidly growing field of microprocessor technology has facilitated the development of this technique, which entails digitalizing and analyzing the reflection of ultrasound waveforms.

Autocorrelation works by matching each incoming waveform with the previous one by repetitively analyzing small segments of the waveforms. In one model of this technique, during a 1.25-second time interval or envelope, 256 slices or digitalized points are taken (one every 5 milliseconds). The 256 points are then compared by means of a mathematical algorithm to the equivalent points obtained in the previous envelope. This process results in rejection of artifactual waveforms and a more accurate identification of the initiation of the fetal cardiac cycle than other techniques provide. Problems with amplitude variations of the waveforms are minimized, and the need for the traditional peak detection is eliminated (Hewlett-Packard, 1984).

All of the monitors that use some form of autocorrelation have technical variations such as the length of time in which waveforms are retained in the memory system and how many waveforms are used for comparison. Further developments and improvements in this technology are ongoing.

Autocorrelation vs. Peak Detection

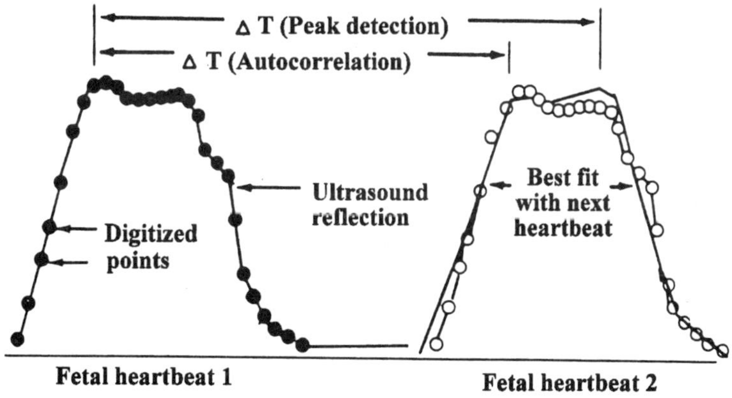

Autocorrelation with peak detection: These two methods differ markedly in how they time heartbeats. Peak detection builds in artificial variability because it cannot pick up at a consistent point on the waveform. Doppler signal processing, with autocorrelation, yields a higher degree of accuracy and permits evaluation of variability.

Figure 2-18. Autocorrelation vs. peak detection (Hewlett-Packard, 1984)

A comparison of the basics of first- and second-generation technology follows (Figure 2-19).

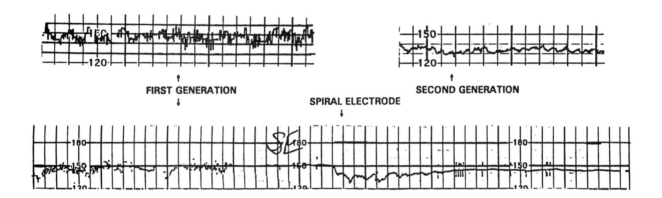

Figure 2-19. Comparison of fetal heart tracings by method used

Doppler Signal Processing

First Generation

- Electronic logic uses peak of waveform as trigger to identify the cardiac event.

- Variable waveforms result in erroneous estimates of short-term or beat-to-beat intervals and produce false variability.

Autocorrelation or
Second Generation

- Electronic logic uses autocorrelation function to identify the cardiac event.

- Microprocessor repetitively analyzes the waveform by comparing multiple points to those of the previous waveform and produces close approximation of short-term variations in the FHR.

<u>Fetal Spiral Electrode</u>

Direct FHR monitoring derives a signal from the fetal electrocardiogram that enables the electronic logic to trigger on the same point in each fetal cardiac cycle---the R wave (Figure 2-20). This process produces a stable tracing and true representation of FHR STV.

<u>Mechanism</u>
- Reproduces FHR by measurement of the interval between R-wave peaks. Each new R-wave arrival recalculates the rate from the previous R-wave interval.

<u>Benefits</u>
- Depicts short-term changes in FHR.
- Allows patients freedom of movement.
- May detect dysrhythmias.

<u>Limitations</u>
- Necessitates rupture of membranes and cervical dilatation.
- Small risk of fetal hemorrhage or infection.
- Electronic interference and artifact may occur.
- Produces a maternal heart rate in the presence of fetal demise.
- Fetal arrhythmias may be missed if the logic or ECG activation switch is on.
- A moist environment is necessary for FHR detection.

INTERPRETATION
SHORT-TERM VARIABILITY

- R-to-R intervals in consecutive QRS complexes to derive FHR
- Internal monitoring
- Fetal reserve
- Parasympathetic nervous system

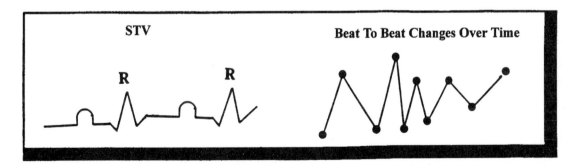

Figure 2-20. Short-term variability detection

Troubleshooting-Instrumentation

The electronic fetal monitor is an instrument which, like any instrument, is capable of equipment malfunction or error. It also is possible that the use of the instrument may be subject to incorrect procedure or human error. Although it is difficult to categorize or list all possible problems, some of them are listed below according to each method or mode of monitoring.

Ultrasound

Problems with the ultrasound (US) may include the following. Erratic recordings or gaps on the tracing paper due to inadequate conduction of the ultrasound signal. Applying ultrasonic gel until a light seal is formed or tightening the ultrasound belt may improve contact and signal accuracy. Fetal or maternal movement also may cause erratic movements. Repositioning the ultrasound transducer or repositioning the mother may improve not only the signal but also the tracing.

An abnormal FHR pattern appearance requires troubleshooting skills. Palpate the mother's pulse and compare it with the audible signal and printed rate to rule out a recording of the maternal pulse. A dysrhythmia also may produce an abnormal FHR pattern. In this case, confirm the FHR by auscultation, preferably with a stethoscope or fetoscope. An abnormal rate printed on the tracing may be caused by doubling or halving by the monitor. This is called "machine halving or machine doubling." The correct rate is established by auscultation. If the circuit integrity of the monitor has been disrupted, press the test button and check the numerical value.

An illegible FHR tracing may be caused by faulty electrical connections or monitor placement. Check the connection to the power source as well as the connections within the monitor. The transducer may be misplaced and may be in need of repositioning. The ultrasound may be repositioned over the fetal back (determined by Leopold's maneuvers), if possible. If the maternal position is a possible source of the problem, reposition the mother. If this does not result in an adequate tracing, try any of the following: Position the ultrasound to face the fetal thorax, position mother laterally, and place ultrasound at the level of the fetal heart in the outer quadrant (just inside the iliac crest bone); if right occiput posterior position or an anterior transverse lie is suspected, try to focus the ultrasound over the fetal back by placing the ultrasound on the maternal back soft tissues. The latter has varying success reports, but when a spiral electrode cannot be placed, it may be worthwhile to try this method. Ultrasound placement is most difficult in maternal obesity, occiput posterior, and anterior wall placenta especially if over the fetal heart. A spiral electrode may be placed when continuous data are needed and cannot be obtained by ultrasound.

Tocodynamometer

Several problems may occur when using the tocodynamometer. If there is no recording on the tracing due to position of the tocodynamometer on the abdomen, palpate the uterus for the area of strongest contraction and reposition the tocodynamometer over that point. Assure that placement of the tocodynamometer is firm, but not tight, on the maternal abdomen. Other problems are illustrated in Figure 2.14. In most cases, repositioning the mother and the tocodynamometer will produce a more accurate tracing of the contractions. Consider using manual palpation to validate uterine activity when the patient is placed laterally and the tocodynamometer is used. If necessary, uterine contractions (UCs) can be indicated on the monitor tracing by using the event or mark buttons on the monitor and/or penned marks.

Spiral Electrode

In addition, several types of problems may occur when using the spiral electrode method of monitoring the fetal heart. There may be intermittent markings on the tracing that could be caused by a failure to detect the electronic activity of the heart; artifact; improperly attached monitor connections; or a fetal dysrhythmia. Solutions for these problems may include the following: Confirm the FHR with a fetoscope; turn off the logic or ECG deactivation switch; test the internal circuitry of the monitor; test the ECG cable and leg plate; check spiral electrode placement, if possible; and apply a new spiral electrode as indicated.

The monitor may display a word such as INOP, to indicate that a signal cannot be received. The leads may not be connected to the leg plate, the spiral electrode (SE) may have a poor connection to the presenting part, or the reference electrode may not be operating. Check the lead connections, gently move the SE wires, and check the EFM circuitry as described. Vaginal secretions may be inadequate and an external reference electrode, if available, may need to be applied.

An electronic signal error may be caused by interference from the maternal signal. If the SE is on the cervix , the maternal signal may be recorded. Confirm the maternal pulse and replace the SE if needed. Manufacturer instruction manuals explain the procedure of separating or distancing the maternal signal from the fetal ECG signal.

The monitor may generate, detect, and print signals other than the FHR. A spiral electrode will record the maternal signal in the presence of a fetal demise. Confirm the maternal pulse when monitoring is initiated or reevaluated. When the pattern appears different from expected, it may be due to paper speed or scaling errors. In this case, verify that the paper speed is adjusted for 3 cm per minute, the preferred speed in the United States and evaluate that paper with proper calibration is being used. Another source of error may be the inability to distinguish artifact from dysrhythmias. Confirm the rate with auscultation, and check all lead connections as previously described.

Intrauterine Pressure Catheter (IUPC)

When using an IUPC to record uterine activity, and there is no recording of contractions, the cause may include displacement of the IUPC, uterine perforation, obstructed catheter, or an incorrectly zeroed IUPC. Troubleshooting includes flushing the fluid filled catheter, zeroing the transducer according to the manufacturer's instructions, and verifying the position of the IUPC. Check the calibration of the transducer if not obtaining any signal. In verifying the position of the IUPC, ask the patient to cough or perform Valsalva's maneuver. If the IUPC is positioned properly, the UC tracing will exhibit a simultaneous spike appearance. If the IUPC has perforated the thinner, lower uterine segment, there may be signs of maternal shock, fetal compromise, failure to record uterine contractions, or an inverse tracing of the UCs.

The uterine resting tone or baseline tonus (5-25 mm Hg) may not be visible due to the need to zero or rezero the IUPC. Rezeroing is accomplished according to the manufacturer's instructions. The uterine resting tone may appear to change as the maternal position changes. This is because the IUPC is sensitive to hydrostatic pressure and changes in hydrostatic pressure. Recording the uterine resting tone in all positions is especially important when using a sensor-tipped IUPC, that cannot be rezeroed after insertion (Figure 2-15).

Fluid-filled IUPCs and sensor-tipped IUPCs which may be rezeroed after insertion, are rezeroed and reevaluated with maternal position changes and as needed. Hospital protocols vary for noting change of shift baseline readings. (Afriat, 1989; Freeman et al., 1991; Hewlett-Packard, 1991; Murray, 1988; Chez & Harvey, 1989; Perlow & Garite, 1991).

When an abnormal appearance of the waveform is noted on the tracing, consider that the end of the IUPC may be lodged against the uterine wall or a fetal body part or that the fluid-filled IUPC may be dry or incompletely filled with sterile water, thus permitting air to dampen the waveform. If this occurs, reposition or flush the IUPC. Twisting the IUPC 180° may change the relationship of the pressure sensing device to the fetus and uterus.

The methods used to assess FHR and uterine activity may change, depending upon the quality of information received for interpretation and the quality of information needed for adequate assessment, interpretation, interventions, and evaluation (Figure 2-21). Changes in the methods of assessment are made to obtain the information needed to adequately assess fetal well-being and uterine activity. The interpretation and nursing diagnosis process begins with the assessment of information. Chapter 3 will continue with interpretation of the FHR characteristics.

Decision Tree for Fetal Heart Monitoring

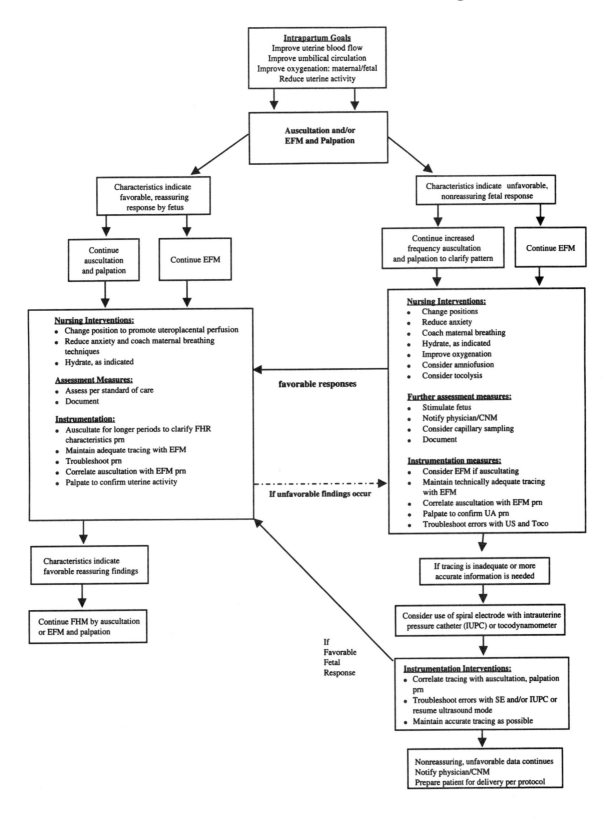

Figure 2-21. This decision tree for selection and verification of instrumentation techniques.

APPENDIX 2a: Assessment: Selected Risk Factors in Pregnancy

Aumann and Baird (1993) suggest further assessment when combinations of the following risk factors are present. This list is not inclusive, and by no means dictates the use of a high-risk pregnancy protocol. The entire assessment process (history, physical findings, testing, etc.), interpretation of data, and response to intervention guide caregivers in providing individualized patient care at the appropriate risk level.

Socioeconomic factors

1. Inadequate finances

2. Poor housing

3. Severe social problems

4. Unwed, especially adolescent

5. Minority status

6. Nutritional deprivation

7. Parental occupation

Demographic Factors

1. Maternal age under 16 or over 35 years

2. Overweight or underweight prior to pregnancy

3. Height less than 5 feet

4. Maternal education less than 11 years

5. Family history of severe inherited disorders

Medical Factors

A. Obstetric History

1. History of infertility

2. Previous ectopic pregnancy or spontaneous abortion

3. Grandmultiparity

4. Previous stillborn or neonatal death

5. Uterine/cervical abnormality

6. Previous multiple gestation

7. Previous premature labor/delivery

8. Previous prolonged labor

9. Previous cesarean section

10. Previous low-birthweight infant

11. Previous macrosomic infant

12. Previous midforceps delivery

13. Previous infant with neurologic deficit, birth injury, or malformation

14. Previous hydatidiform mole or choriocarcinoma

B. Maternal Medical History/Status

1. Maternal cardiac disease

2. Maternal pulmonary disease

3. Maternal metabolic disease (particularly diabetes mellitus or thyroid disease)

4. Chronic renal disease, repeated urinary tract infection, repeated bacteriuria

5. Maternal gastrointestinal disease

6. Maternal endocrine disorders (pituitary, adrenal)

7. Chronic hypertension

8. Maternal hemoglobinopathies

9. Seizure disorder

10. Venereal and other infectious diseases

11. Weight loss greater than 5 lbs

12. Malignancy

13. Surgery during pregnancy

14. Major congenital anomalies of the reproductive tract

15. Maternal mental retardation, major emotional disorders

C. Current Obstetric Status

1. Late or no prenatal care

2. Rh sensitization

3. Fetus inappropriately large or small for gestation

4. Premature labor

5.   Pregnancy-induced hypertension

6.   Multiple gestation

7.   Polyhydramnios

8.   Premature rupture of the membranes

9.   Antepartum bleeding

   a. Placenta previa

   b. Abruptio placenta

10.   Abnormal presentation

11.   Postmaturity

12.   Abnormality in test for fetal well-being

13.   Maternal anemia

D. Habits/Habituation

1.   Smoking during pregnancy

2.   Regular alcohol intake

3.   Drug use/abuse

REFERENCES

American Academy of Pediatrics and American College of Obstetricians and Gynecologists (AAP & ACOG). (1992). Guidelines for Perinatal Care (3rd ed.). Elk Grove Village, IL: Author.

American College of Obstetricians and Gynecologists (ACOG). (1989a). Intrapartum fetal heart rate monitoring, ACOG Technical Bulletin No. 132. Washington, DC: Author.

American College of Obstetricians and Gynecologists (ACOG). (1989b). Standards for obstetric-gynecologic services (7th ed.). Washington, DC: Author.

American College of Obstetricians and Gynecologists (ACOG). (1995). Fetal heart rate patterns: Monitoring, interpretation, and management, ACOG Technical Bulletin No. 207. Washington, DC: Author.

Association of Women's Health, Obstetric and Neonatal Nurses (AWHONN). (1992). Nursing responsibilities in implementing intrapartum fetal heart rate monitoring. Position Statement. Washington, DC: Author.

Afriat, C. (1989). Electronic fetal monitoring. Rockville, MD: Aspen Publications.

Aumann, G. M., & Baird, M. M. (1993). Risk assessment for pregnant women. In R.A. Knuppel & J. E. Drukker (Eds.), High risk pregnancy: A team approach (2nd ed.) (p.13). Philadelphia: W. B. Saunders Company.

Bernardes, J. (1996). Efficacy and safety of intrapartum electronic fetal monitoring: An update (Letter). Obstetrics and Gynecology, 87, 476.

Bissonnette, J. (1991). Placental and fetal physiology. In S. Gabbe, J. Niebyl, & J. Simpson (Eds.), Obstetrics: Normal and problem pregnancies (2nd ed.) (p. 93). New York: Churchill Livingstone.

Bobak, I. M., Jensen, M. D., & Zalar, M. K. (1989). Maternity and gynecologic care: The nurse and the family (4th ed.). St. Louis: C. V. Mosby Company.

Boehm, F., Fields, L., Hutchison, J., Bowen, A. W., & Vaughn, W. K. (1986). The indirectly obtained fetal heart rate: Comparison of first and second generation electronic fetal monitors. American Journal of Obstetrics and Gynecology, 155(1), 10-14.

Caldeyro-Barcia, R., & Poseiro, J. J. (1960). Physiology of the uterine contraction. Clinical Obstetrics and Gynecology, 3, 386-408.

Clark, S. (1990). How a modified NST improves fetal surveillance. Contemporary OB/GYN, 35(5), 45-48.

Chez, B. F., & Harvey, C. (1989). Critical concepts in fetal heart rate monitoring. Videotape series: Association of Women's Health, Obstetric and Neonatal Nurses (AWHONN). Baltimore, MD: Williams and Wilkins.

Freeman, R. K., & Garite, T. J. (1981). Fetal heart rate monitoring. Baltimore: Williams and Wilkins.

Freeman, R. K., Garite, T. J., & Nageotte, M. P. (1991). Fetal heart rate monitoring (2nd ed.). Baltimore: Williams and Wilkins.

Hewlett-Packard. (1984). The technology within. Andover, MA: Author.

Hewlett-Packard. (1991). Manufacturer's instructions for model 1350A. Andover, MA: Author.

Heymann, M. (1989). Fetal cardiovascular physiology. In R. K. Creasy & R. Resnik (Eds.), Maternal fetal medicine: Principles and practice (2nd ed.) (p. 288). Philadelphia: W. B. Saunders Company.

Hon, E. H. (1975). An introduction to fetal heart rate monitoring (2nd ed.). Los Angeles: USC School of Medicine.

Hutson, J., & Petrie, R. (1986). Possible limitations of fetal monitoring. Clinical Obstetrics and Gynecology, 29,(1) 104-113.

Itskovitz, J., La Gamma, E. F., & Rudolph, A. M. (1983). Heart rate and blood pressure responses to umbilical cord compression in fetal lambs with special reference to the mechanism of variable deceleration. American Journal of Obstetrics and Gynecology, 147(4), 451-457.

James, L. S., Yeh, M. N., Morishima, H. O., Daniel, S. S., Cartiis, S. N., Niemann, W. H., & Indyk, L. (1976). Umbilical vein occlusion and transient acceleration of the fetal heart. American Journal of Obstetrics and Gynecology, 126(2), 276-283.

Jensen, M. D., Benson, R. C., & Bobak, I. M. (1981). Maternity care: The nurse and the family (2nd ed.). St. Louis: Mosby Company.

Kirkinen, P., Jouppila, P., Koivula, A., Vuori, J., & Puukka, M. (1983). The effect of caffeine on placental and fetal blood flow in human pregnancy. American Journal of Obstetrics and Gynecology, 147(8), 939-942.

Klapholz, H. (1978). Techniques of fetal heart monitoring. Seminars in Perinatology, 2(2), 1.

Klavan, M., Laver, A. T., & Boscola, M. (1977). Clinical concepts of fetal heart rate monitoring. Andover, MA: Hewlett-Packard Company.

Lagercrantz, H., & Slotkin, T. (1986). The "stress" of being born. Scientific American, 254(4), 100-107.

Malinowski, J. S., Pedigo, C. G., & Phillips, C. R. (1989). Nursing care during the labor process (3rd ed.). Philadelphia: F. A. Davis Company.

Maygrier, J. P. (1834). Midwifery illustrated. New York: Harper & Brothers. Facsimile Edition 1969, by Medical Heritage Press, Inc., Skokie, IL.

McCusker, J., Harris, D. R., & Hosmer, D. W. (1988). Association of electronic fetal monitoring during labor with cesarean section rate and with neonatal morbidity and mortality. American Journal of Public Health, 78(9), 1170-1174.

Meschia, G. (1985). Safety margin of fetal oxygenation. Journal of Reproductive Medicine, 30,(4)308-311.

Meschia, G. (1989). Placental respiratory gas exchange and fetal oxygenation. In R. K. Creasy & R. Resnik (Eds.), Maternal fetal medicine: Principles and practice (2nd ed.). Philadelphia: W. B. Saunders Company.

Moore, K.L. (1993). The developing human (2nd ed.). Philadelphia: W.B. Saunders Company.

Morrison, J., Chez, B., Davis, I., Martin, R., Roberts, W., Martin, J., & Floyd, R. (1993). Intrapartum fetal heart assessment: Monitoring by auscultation or electronic means. American Journal of Obstetrics and Gynecology, 168 (1), 63-66.

Murray, M. (1988). Antepartum and intrapartum fetal monitoring. Washington, DC: NAACOG.

NAACOG. (1990). Fetal heart rate auscultation, OGN Nursing Practice Resource. Washington, DC: Author.

NAACOG. (1991). Standards of intrapartum nursing practice. In NAACOG standards for the nursing care of women and newborns (4th ed.) (pp.34-39). Washington, DC: Author.

Olds, S., London, M., & Ladewig, P. (1992). Maternal-newborn nursing: A family centered approach (4th Ed.). Menlo Park, CA: Addison-Wesley Publishing.

Oxorn, H. (1986). Oxorn-Foote: Human labor and birth (5th ed.). Norwalk, CT: Appleton-Century-Crofts.

Paine, L. (1992). A comparison of the auscultated acceleration test and the nonstress test as predictors of perinatal outcomes. Nursing Research, 41 (2), 87-91.

Parer, J. T. (1976). Physiologic effect of fetal heart rate. Journal of Obstetric, Gynecologic, and Neonatal Nursing, 5(Suppl. 5), 27s.

Parer, J. T. (1983a). Fetal cardiorespiratory physiology. In Handbook of fetal heart rate monitoring. Philadelphia: W. B. Saunders Company.

Parer, J. T. (1983b). Uteroplacental physiology and exchange. In Handbook of fetal heart rate monitoring (p. 15). Philadelphia: W. B. Saunders Company.

Parer, J. T. (1989). Fetal heart rate. In R. K. Creasy & R. Resnik (Eds.), Maternal fetal medicine: Principles and practice (p. 314). Philadelphia: W. B. Saunders Company

Parer, J. T. (1994). Fetal heart rate. In R.K. Creasy & R. Resnik (Eds.), Maternal fetal medicine, (3rd ed.) (298-325). Philadelphia: W.B. Saunders Company.

Parer, J.T. (1996). Efficacy and safety of intrapartum electronic fetal monitoring: An update (Letter). Obstetrics and Gynecology, 87, 476-477.

Perlow, J. H., & Garite, T. J. (1991). Update on electronic fetal monitoring systems. Contemporary OB/GYN, 36(Suppl.), 44.

Phelan, J. (1989). The postdate pregnancy: An overview. Clinical Obstetrics and Gynecology, 32(2), 221.

Poseiro, J. J. (1969). Effect of uterine contractions on maternal blood flow through the placenta. In Perinatal factors affecting human development (p. 161-171). Pan American Health Organization, Pub. #185.

Simpson, K., & Creehan, P. (1996). Perinatal nursing. Philadelphia: Lippincott-Raven Publishers/Washington, DC: AWHONN.

Snydal, S. H. (1988). Methods of fetal heart rate monitoring during labor. A selective review of the literature. Journal of Nurse-Midwifery, 33(1), 4-14.

Society of Obstetricians and Gynaecologists of Canada (SOGC). (1995). SOGC Policy Statement: Fetal health surveillance in labour. Journal of SOGC, 17(9), 865-901.

Strong, T. H., & Paul, R. H. (1989). Intrapartum uterine activity: Evaluation of an intrauterine pressure transducer. Obstetrics and Gynecology, 73(3.1), 432-434.

Supplee, R. B., & Vezeau, T. M. (1996). Continuous electronic fetal monitoring: Does it belong in low-risk births? Maternal Child Nursing, 21, 301-306.

Thacker, S.B., & Stroup, D.F. (1996). Efficacy and safety of intrapartum electronic fetal monitoring: An update (Letter). Obstetrics and Gynecology, 87, 477.

Thacker, S.B., Stroup, D.F., & Peterson, H.B. (1995). Efficacy and safety of intrapartum electronic fetal monitoring: An update. Obstetrics and Gynecology, 86, 613-620.

Vintzeleos, A.M., Nochimson, D.J., Antsaklis, A., Varvarigos, I., Guzman, E.R., & Knuppel, R.A. (1995). Comparison of intrapartum electronic fetal heart rate monitoring versus intermittent auscultation in detecting fetal acidemia at birth. American Journal of Obstetrics and Gynecology, 173, 1021-1024.

Vintzileos, A.M., Nochimson, D.J., Guzman, E.R., Knuppel, R. A., Lake, M., & Schrifrin, B.S. (1995). Intrapartum electronic fetal heart rate monitoring versus intermittent auscultation: A meta-analysis. Obstetrics & Gynecology, 85(1), 149-155.

Vintzileos, A.M., Antsaklis, A., Varvarigos, I., Papas, C., Sofatzis, I., & Montgomer, J.T. (1993). A randomized trial of intrapartum electronic fetal heart monitoring versus intermittent auscultation. Obstetrics & Gynecology, 81(6), 899-907.

Zuspan, F. P., O'Shaughnessy, R., & Iams, J. D. (1981). The role of the adrenal gland and sympathetic nervous system in pregnancy. Journal of Reproductive Medicine, 26(9), 483-491.

BIBLIOGRAPHY

Bieniarz, J., Branda, L. A., Maqueda, E., Morozovsky, J., & Caldeyro-Barcia, R. (1968). Aortocaval compression by the uterus in late pregnancy. Unreliability of the sphygmomanometric method in estimating uterine artery pressure. American Journal of Obstetrics and Gynecology, 102(8), 1106-1115.

Bobak, I. M., & Jensen, M. D. (1991). Essentials of maternity nursing, (3rd ed.). St. Louis: C. V. Mosby Company.

Copper, R. L., & Goldenberg, R. L. (1990). Catecholamine secretion in fetal adaptation to stress. Journal of Obstetric, Gynecologic, and Neonatal Nursing, 19(3), 223-226.

Harvey, C., & Chez, B. F. (1996). Critical concepts in fetal heart rate monitoring (2nd ed.). Videotape series: Association of Women's Health, Obstetric and Neonatal Nurses (AWHONN). Baltimore, MD: Williams and Wilkins.

Leveno, K. J., Cunningham, F. G., Nelson, S., Roark, M., Williams, M. L., Guzick, D., Dowling, S., Rosenfeld, C. R., & Buckley, A. (1986). A prospective comparison of selective and universal electronic fetal monitoring in 34,995 pregnancies. New England Journal of Medicine, 315(10), 615-619.

Spence, A. P., & Mason, E. B. (1987). Human anatomy and physiology. Menlo Park, CA: Benjamin/Cummings.

Tucker, S. (1992). Pocket guide to fetal monitoring (2nd ed.). St. Louis: Mosby Year Book.

Wagner, P. C., Cabaniss, M. L., & Johnson, T. R. B. (1985). What's really new in EFM equipment? Contemporary OB/GYN, 26(Suppl.), 96.

Wilson, R. W., & Schifrin, B. S. (1980). Is any pregnancy low risk? Obstetrics and Gynecology, 55(5), 653-656.

CHAPTER 3: INTERPRETATION

Introduction

This chapter provides concepts for nursing process interpretation of FHR characteristics (Figure 3-1). Interpretation includes the systematic analysis of collected assessment data necessary for collaborative diagnosis and intervention. Emphasis is placed on the physiologic basis of FHR characteristics found on electronic fetal monitoring tracings.

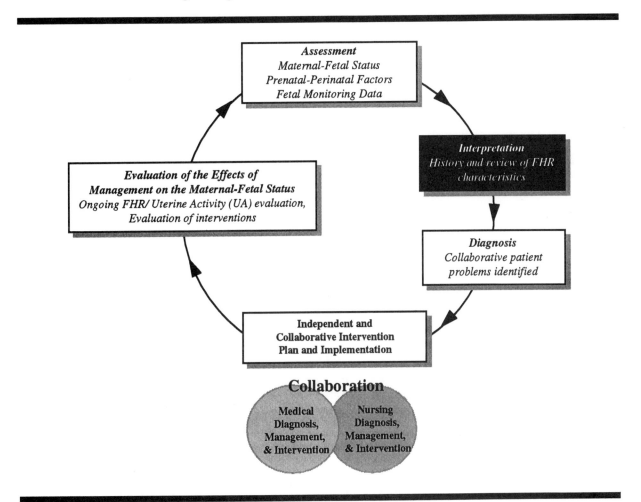

Figure 3-1. The nursing process and fetal heart monitoring: Interpretation.

Much of the technology developed to improve perinatal outcomes focuses on indirect measures of fetal status because a direct examination of the fetus is difficult. During the last three decades, the most useful, yet controversial, techniques have centered around the evaluation of the fetal heart. Whether auscultated or electronically monitored, the fetal heart is the element that is most easily and frequently observed in fetal evaluation. The electronic fetal monitor is a piece of equipment that obtains the FHR and monitors uterine activity continuously and easily. The monitor provides assessment data to be used in much the same way as an automatic blood pressure cuff and pulse device, or even a hemodynamic monitor.

Health-care providers who use EFM will benefit most by knowing whether the data generated is valid. Also the focus is not only upon the data the monitor provides, but also on the physiologic status the data implies. Such a focus will help improve interpretation. The uninformed and unwary practitioner may misinterpret impressive-appearing patterns without adequate knowledge of related physiologic status.

Practitioners involved with interpreting FHR monitoring tracings agree on one aspect—that there is a lack of agreed upon, reproducible definitions or terminology in clinical trials and clinical practice. That inconsistency challenges even the fetal monitoring experts. Regardless of practice setting, the process of interpreting an FHR monitoring tracing includes a) examining the tracing for trends of all FHR and uterine activity parameters and b) answering the question "At the present time, what is the likely status of this fetus?" In light of all that is presented in the literature, it is important to realize that FHR monitoring is but one parameter of fetal well-being and is not a substitute for informed clinical judgment (ACOG, 1995b; SOGC, 1995).

It also is important to consider that the interpretation of FHR tracings is difficult enough without the added factor of prematurity. Interpreting preterm FHR tracings requires an astute knowledge of fetal development and its underlying physiologic changes. This section also will provide some insight into the interpretation of the preterm FHR tracing.

Various physiologic events may affect uterine or uteroplacental blood flow to the fetus and reduce fetal oxygen supply. The fetus may tolerate decreased uterine or umbilical blood flow for a time and even compensate using changes in the FHR. During such times, the FHR may indicate physiologic stress; however, the fetus also may continue to demonstrate reassuring factors of fetal well-being, such as the presence of variability.

At other times, the oxygen may fall below the critical level needed by the fetus. The FHR shows nonreassuring signs of fetal well-being in these situations. Often it is difficult to determine whether the onset of fetal compromise and nonreassuring pattern has occurred prior to or during labor.

Health-care providers use clinical data about the fetal status to plan interventions to promote or maintain fetal well-being, lessen the physiologic stress, or correct and improve nonreassuring symptoms. A pattern type often can be described as either reassuring or nonreassuring. Recognizing the fetal need for some type of intervention becomes important as nonreassuring patterns develop.

Specific changes in physiology, especially during the dynamic intrapartum period, precipitate characteristic FHR patterns. When these characteristic FHR patterns are observed, one usually assumes that a related physiologic event is simultaneously present. With awareness of the event and its severity, health care providers may make more knowledgeable decisions. A systematic assessment of the fetal heart, with emphasis on its physiologic basis, will provide data to evaluate fetal well-being and assist with overall maternal-fetal management (Figure 3-1). As the systematic assessment is discussed in the following pages, the table below is progressively developed, highlighting and depicting each classification and subclassification. First, the baseline fetal heart characteristics of rate, variability, and rhythm will be addressed. This will be followed by a discussion of fetal heart changes from the base line, including accelerations and decelerations.

Baseline	Fetal Heart Changes	
Rate		
Normal	Periodic	Nonperiodic
Tachycardia		
Bradycardia	Accelerations	Accelerations
	Decelerations	Decelerations
Variability	Variable	Variable
STV	Late	Prolonged
LTV	Early	
Undulating	Combined deceleration patterns	
Rhythm		
Regular		
Irregular		

Baseline Rate

Baseline	Fetal Heart Changes
RATE Normal Tachycardia Bradycardia	

Today, the commonly accepted normal baseline rate is 110-160 bpm (Murray, 1996; Simpson & Creehan, 1996; SOGC, 1995; Tucker, 1996). In the past, the accepted normal baseline FHR was 120-160 beats per minute (bpm) (ACOG, 1995b; Freeman, Garite, & Nageotte, 1991; Hon, 1975; Klavan, Laver, & Boscola, 1977; Parer, 1989; Paul, Petrie, Rabello, & Mueller, 1985; Petrie, 1991; Simpkin, 1986; Tucker, 1992). FHRs between 110 and 120 are often considered as normal in fetuses over age 40 weeks of gestation (ACOG, 1995b; Simpson & Creehan, 1996; SOGC, 1995). The normal fetal baseline heart rate can be obtained via auscultation, ultrasound, or spiral electrode methods. For a discussion of these methods, refer to Techniques of Fetal Heart Monitoring, beginning in Chapter 2 of this manual.

Generally a baseline is established by assessing the FHR for a minimum of 10 minutes to observe a sustained rate. Variations from the normal baseline rate are called *tachycardia* and *bradycardia*.

Tachycardia

Tachycardia is defined by many authorities as an FHR above 160 bpm for at least 10 minutes. The causes of tachycardia can be traced most often to maternal fever or to infection in the mother, fetus, or both. Although the preterm heart rate may be toward the upper range of normal, the heart rate of a preterm fetus usually does not exceed 160 bpm. The care provider may notice a slight but gradual decrease of the FHR baseline as gestational age increases. Tachycardia represents increased sympathetic and decreased parasympathetic autonomic tone and, due to this control, is generally associated with loss of FHR baseline variability (Freeman et al., 1991). It also is important to watch for a gradual increase in the FHR that can occur over time, even before the FHR exceeds 160 bpm. Further assessment of the fetus with baseline tachycardia includes evaluation of variability (long- and short-term), reactivity, decelerations, and the duration of the observed pattern (Figure 3-2). When tachycardia persists over 200 bpm, fetal hydrops or demise may occur. More information on this type of pattern is contained in a discussion of rhythm later in this section. The fetus may or may not demonstrate variability for a period of time with mild tachycardia of 160-180 bpm. This also is associated with a dominance of the sympathetic nervous system (SNS) over the parasympathetic nervous system (PSNS). The interaction between the SNS and the PSNS is necessary to produce short-term variability (STV).

Causes of Tachycardia

Maternal

- fever
- infection
- dehydration
- hyperthyroidism
- endogenous adrenaline/anxiety
- medication or drug response
  (e.g., betasympathomimetic
  agents, parasympatholytics,
  inotropic, drugs, illicit drugs)
- anemia

Fetal

- infection
- prolonged fetal activity or stimulation
- compensatory effort following hypoxemia
- chronic hypoxemia
- cardiac abnormalities, heart failure
- supraventricular tachycardia
- prematurity
- congenital anomalies

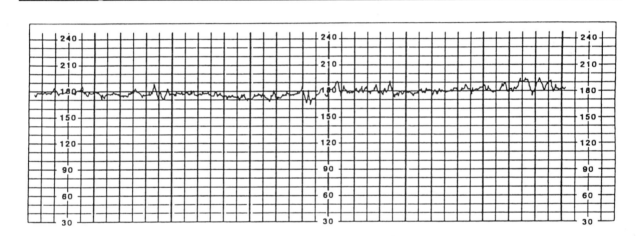

Figure 3-2. Example of tachycardia. This FHR tracing shows a baseline rate of 175-185 bpm with average LTV.

Bradycardia

When the FHR is below 110-120 bpm for at least 10 minutes, a condition called bradycardia is present (Figure 3-3). Bradycardia, present when the heart rate is between 100-120 bpm (Parer, 1989), or even 90-120 bpm (Freeman et al., 1991), often demonstrates adequate LTV and STV. Adequate variability is much less likely to be present when the FHR persists below 90 bpm for more than 10 minutes. If there is variability present with bradycardia, the bradycardia can be considered benign/reassuring (Freeman et al., 1991). The inability of the fetus to alter its cardiac output significantly increases the likelihood of an inadequate oxygen level at the lower heart rate. The lower the heart rate, the lower the cardiac output. An exception is complete heart block, which has a typical fetal rate of 60-80 bpm and may be associated with normal oxygenation. Complete heart block often is associated with clinical or serologic evidence of maternal collagen vascular disease, especially systemic lupus erythematosus

(Hohn & Stanton, 1992; Tucker, 1992). Bradycardia is evaluated in conjunction with FHR variability, reactivity, and the severity and persistence of the bradycardia. Differentiating between a persistent bradycardic rate and a prolonged deceleration also helps to evaluate fetal status. It also is important to differentiate between fetal and maternal heart rates when a persistent bradycardic rate is observed.

Causes of Bradycardia

Maternal	Fetal
- position	- may occur with mature parasympathetic nervous system (PSNS)
- hypotension	
- drug responses	- umbilical cord occlusion (e.g., prolapsed cord)
- connective tissue disease, for example, systemic lupus erythematosus (SLE)	- decompensated fetus
	- hypothermia
	- cardiac conduction defect
- prolonged maternal hypoglycemia	- cardiac structural defect
	- excessive PSNS tone produced by chronic head compression in a vertex presentation, occiput posterior, or transverse position (vagal stimulation)

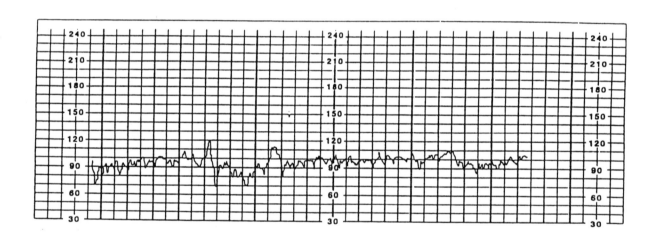

Figure 3-3. Example of bradycardia. This tracing demonstrates a baseline rate of 90 to 100 bpm with average LTV per ultrasound EFM.

Variability

Baseline	Fetal Heart Changes

Rate
   Normal
   Tachycardia
   Bradycardia
 	
VARIABILITY	

Variability is the term used to characterize the baseline FHR variations from beat-to-beat (STV) and changes over 1 minute time intervals (LTV). It represents the interplay and balance between the sympathetic (cardioaccelerator) and parasympathetic (cardiodecelerator) divisions of the autonomic nervous system. Variability is largely controlled by the autonomic nervous system and reflects central nervous system (CNS) status. Therefore, variability is the single most important characteristic of the FHR. Variability is discussed as a single term, but actually refers to both LTV and STV.

Physiology of Variability

Variability is derived from impulses of the medulla's sympathetic and parasympathetic nervous systems. Nerve fibers from these systems innervate the myocardium and the sinoatrial (SA) and atrioventricular (AV) nodes, respectively (Figure 2-2). The status of the brain stem's medulla oblongata, therefore, controls nerve fiber innervation to the heart. It is appropriate to discuss the assorted influences on the medulla oblongata. Influences that alter variability via the medulla are oxygenation status, cardiac output regulation, fetal behavior during sleep and awake states, hormonal regulation, and drug effects (Freeman et al., 1991; Martin, 1982; Parer, 1989; Petrie, 1991). Normal variability of the FHR is a reflection of an intact neurologic modulation of the FHR, normal cardiac responsiveness, and fetal reserve (Freeman et al., 1991; Rosen & Dickinson, 1993; Tucker, 1992).

The influences on variability and rate often interrelate. For example, a transient central hypoxemia may stimulate chemoreceptors which increase catecholamines, variability oscillation appearance, and peripheral vascular resistance; cardiac output improves, thereby improving blood flow to the brain, heart, and adrenal glands. The variability oscillations then revert to average or within normal limits. In this example, the presence of variability (LTV and STV) represents an intact neuromodulation of the FHR and normal cardiac responsiveness. Variability may increase with fetal breathing, hemodynamic changes, and may increase or decrease with sleep states. The quiet sleep state elicits fewer variability cycles, and the rapid eye movement (REM) sleep state elicits more variability (Martin, 1982). Emotional states may be integrated into the CNS via the hypothalamus and sympathetic response exhibiting changes in variability oscillations, blood pressure, baroreflex, and heart rate (Parer, 1989). An anencephalic or hydrocephalic fetus without an intact medulla will exhibit minimal and absent variability regardless of fetal oxygenation state.

Key points on variability include the following:

- Oxygenation of the central nervous system influences impulse transmission of the FHR.
- Adequate oxygenation and an intact autonomic nervous system contribute to creating variability (LTV and STV).
- Absent or decreased variability may be due to alterations in nervous system function or inadequate oxygenation, or both.
- Alterations of the nervous system function are associated with fetal sleep and wake states, medications, alcohol, and illicit drugs, or anomalies that may alter the variability.
- Oxygenation compromise may alter the variability.

Types of Variability

Baseline	Fetal Heart Changes
Rate 　Normal 　Tachycardia 　Bradycardia **VARIABILITY** 　**STV** 　**LTV** 　**UNDULATING**	

Short-Term Variability (STV)

Within the autonomic nervous system, the PSNS has a greater influence on variability, especially STV. The parasympathetic influences occur much more rapidly than the sympathetic influence and are responsible for fine-tuning the fetal heart's STV. The comparative sympathetic response time lag is 2-3 seconds, and the return to baseline is even slower (Martin, 1982). When the medulla is hypoxic, poor impulse transmission occurs. The poor transmission usually causes a loss of STV first, followed by minimal LTV. STV is believed to be an important prognostic indicator of fetal outcome.

STV Assessment

With a spiral electrode placed on the fetus, STV can be assessed. STV reflects changes in the FHR from one beat to the next beat. Even though only a time interval between two beats is measured and computed, the number value represents a presumed 1 minute rate. Often the question arises regarding autocorrelation with external monitors. All monitors today use some form of autocorrelation. Autocorrelation rejects most artifact waveforms, which may improve the appearance of the tracing, but does not guarantee the presence of STV.

The R-to-R interval of the QRS complex of the fetal cardiac cycle is measured in milliseconds, and this constant change causes the line of the FHR tracing to appear "rough" and/or "squiggly," indicating the tiny increases and decreases in the rate. Because this short-term interval is changing constantly in the healthy fetus, the numbers change continuously on the digital display of the monitor. It is difficult to numerically quantify the changes visualized on the tracing into levels or degrees. Due to the rapid nature of these changes, the only accurate way to adequately assess STV is with internal, continuous fetal monitoring (ACOG, 1995; May & Mahlmeister, 1994).

Regardless of the many ways used to describe STV, the most practical way is to determine the presence or absence of STV. This is done by examining the characteristics of the fetal heart tracing line and assessing the tracing for roughness or smoothness (Figure 3-4). The term present may be used to denote roughness of the tracing line, and the term absent may be used to denote smoothness of the tracing line (Figure 3-4).

STV Characteristics

- Measured as the variation in time intervals between R waves of each cardiac cycle.
- Interpreted as present or absent with the spiral electrode.
- Controlled by PSNS.

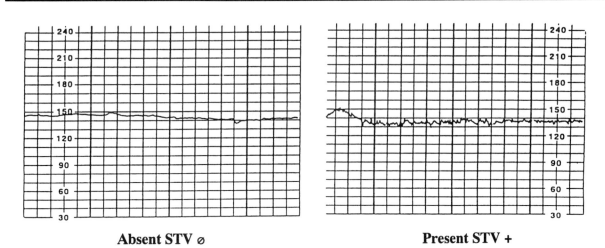

Absent STV ⊘   **Present STV +**

The first tracing depicts a fetus with absent STV. The second tracing depicts a fetus with present STV.

Figure 3-4. Example of absent and present STV.

Long-term variability (LTV)

LTV is a characteristic of baseline fetal heart rate and does not include accelerations or decelerations. LTV is characterized by fluctuations or oscillations in the FHR, described as cycles per minute. The cycles portray the amplitude or rise and fall of the heart rate within its baseline range (Figures 3-5, 3-6, 3-7, and 3-8). The frequency of the fluctuations of LTV can be determined by counting a) the number of complete cycles per minute, b) the number of turning points, or c) the number of crossings over an imaginary line within 1 minute (Martin, 1982; Petrie, 1991).

LTV Categories

Different categories have been used to describe LTV. Each category defines a range of change in the heart rate from its baseline in bpm. Because this deviation from the baseline FHR is expressed in bpm, it is referred to as the amplitude. Consensus has yet to be achieved across the fetal monitoring community on categories of variability. As a means to standardize terminology for this course, three levels of LTV amplitude are presented: decreased or minimal, 0-5 bpm; average or within normal limits, 6-25 bpm; or marked or saltatory, > 25 bpm. Categories of these terms and appropriate abbreviations are represented in Figure 3-8.

Average or Within Normal Limits

Average LTV values of the FHR amplitude are described as 6-25 bpm, and the frequency of fluctuations or cycles as 3-6 per minute (Hammacher, 1969; Martin, 1982; Parer, 1989; Simpson & Creehan, 1996). The fetal wake state, behavioral state, and responsiveness result in variations within this relatively wide average range.

Decreased or Minimal

Interventions indicated for a persistent decrease in LTV, whether 0-2 bpm or 3-5 bpm range, usually are the same. It is, therefore, clinically appropriate to consider 0-5 bpm change as a single category. Such a persistent pattern of decreased FHR variability in the absence of medication or known anomalies requires some form of intervention and physician or midwife notification. When the duration of the pattern is beyond a fetal sleep cycle and the FHR remains nonreactive to stimulation, further nursing assessments and interventions should be considered. Fetal behavioral states alone can have a tremendous influence on variability. While more than 50% of fetal sleep cycles will last less than 40 minutes, it is known that some fetuses will have sleep cycles lasting 80-90 minutes or more. Prior to initiating all interventions with the onset of decreased variability, it is appropriate to review and evaluate the fetal heart response, behavioral state, response to stimulation, and the total clinical picture (e.g., medications, narcotics, anomalies).

Marked or Saltatory

Marked LTV etiology is uncertain even though it is noted to be primarily an intrapartum pattern (Parer, 1989; Petrie, 1991). It is noted that the fetus is likely exhibiting a sympathetic response to brief, acute periods of hypoxemia. Attempts to resolve a marked or saltatory pattern are appropriate (see Chapter 4 Interventions).

Interpretation of FHR Variability

Variability (LTV and STV) provides useful information as to the status of the fetus. There are significant factors to consider in the interpretation of LTV and STV. These factors may include the following:

1. The instrumentation used to obtain the signal will dictate the parameters which can be assessed (ACOG, 1995b; Martin, 1982; Parer, 1983; Rosen & Dickinson, 1993). For example, when using ultrasound, baseline FHR and LTV can be interpreted. When using the spiral electrode, not only the baseline FHR and LTV, but also the STV, can be interpreted.

2. The presence of STV usually indicates a well-oxygenated, nonacidotic fetus.

3. Average LTV may indicate an awake, active fetus responding to the environment.

4. Generally LTV and STV change simultaneously. However, there are times when one may or may not be present with the other. There are times when STV is absent and LTV is present (e.g., sinusoidal or undulating patterns) and conversely when LTV is decreased and STV is present (e.g., a sleeping fetus).

5. A smooth baseline FHR (without variability) may be the result of hypoxemia or a central nervous system anomaly.

6. Decreased LTV may occur temporarily when the fetus is in a sleep cycle.

7. Presence of FHR variability with deceleration patterns indicates the presence of fetal reserve. The insult may be mild and/or of recent origin (Martin, 1982).

8. Decreased variability of the FHR in combination with late or variable decelerations may imply impending acidemia or hypoxemia requiring further assessment.

9. The following questions may assist with interpretations:

   - Was the fetus previously active and was LTV within normal limits?

   - Could the fetus be in a temporary sleep pattern?

   - If STV can be evaluated, is it present?

   - Does the fetus respond to stimuli?

As implied, interpretation includes consideration of actual FHM data as well as other assessment data.

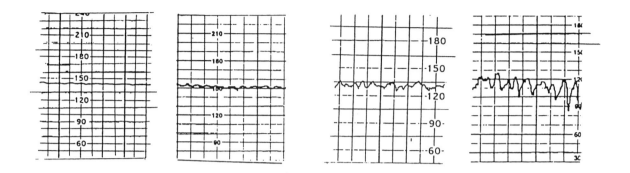

Figure 3-5. Two examples of decreased or minimal LTV.

Figure 3-6. Two examples demonstrating fetuses with average or within normal limits LTV.

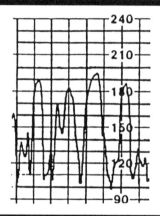

Figure 3-7. This fetus is exhibiting marked or saltatory LTV.

LTV Interpretation

Abbreviation	Variation of Baseline Range	Descriptive Term
LTV ⇓	0 - 5 bpm	Decreased or Minimal
LTV +	6 - 25 bpm	Average or Within Normal Limits
LTV ⇑	> 25 bpm	Marked or Saltatory

Figure 3-8. An example of interpretation of LTV using a three-category system.

Undulating Patterns

Undulating variations in the FHR baseline are known to have a characteristic repetitive shape, resembling a sine wave. Even though the pattern is distinctive, the rate usually is within normal range. These shapes are often described as either <u>sinusoidal</u> or <u>pseudosinusoidal</u> and are sometimes difficult to differentiate from each other. Hence, the word <u>undulating</u> describes the characteristic shape of the wave and is applied when one cannot visually distinguish sinusoidal from pseudosinusoidal waves.

As the name *sinusoidal* suggests, the sinusoidal pattern resembles a sine wave or uniform wavelike undulations that occur above and below an arbitrarily fixed baseline and appear as copies of themselves. When the pattern is smooth, uniform, and persistent, it is sinusoidal and is thought to be serious (Figure 3-9). The less smooth and less constant type of undulating pattern, which appears temporarily following maternal analgesic administration, is thought to be benign and is often called *pseudosinusoidal*. In addition to unequal oscillations above and below the baseline, normal STV and fetal reactivity may be present (Figure 3-10). This pattern has been described as appearing "sawtoothed."

When either pattern is observed, the caregiver always must consider the events that have been associated with sinusoidal patterns.

Characteristics of Sinusoidal Patterns

- Persistent oscillating pattern: 120-160 bpm (sine wave).
- Amplitude of undulations is usually 5-15 bpm.
- Frequency of undulations is usually 2-5 cycles per minute.
- Absent STV.
- Undulating pattern that precludes any other definition of LTV.
- No fetal accelerations, even in response to fetal movement.
- Absence of specific response to uterine contractions.

Events Associated with a Sinusoidal Pattern

- Rh isoimmunization.
- Severe fetal anemia.
- Abruptio placentae.
- Severe fetal acidosis.
- Fetal-maternal hemorrhage.

Characteristics of Pseudosinusoidal Patterns

- "Saw-toothed" appearances.
- Less uniform oscillations.
- Periods of normal variability (LTV, STV).
- Accelerations may be present.

Events Associated With Pseudosinusoidal Patterns

- Narcotic administration or ingestion.
- Analgesic administration.
- Thumb sucking of fetus.
- Unknown, other mitigating circumstances.

Further Considerations for Undulating Fetal Patterns

- Apply a spiral electrode if indicated.
- Assess all monitor data for area of normal baseline.
- Assess maternal-fetal history to identify the fetus at risk (e.g., for anemia).
- Notify physician or midwife.
- Ultrasonography for hydropic appearance.
- Kleihauer-Betke test on maternal serum or APT test of vaginal blood to detect fetal red blood cells.
- Prepare for prompt delivery and expert neonatal care or transport to level III facility.

Other events that have been documented in association with undulating patterns are postdate pregnancy, meconium aspiration, diabetes, and preeclampsia. The literature also reports that sinusoidal patterns due to anemia have been reversed following administration of fetal transfusion or post delivery neonatal exchange transfusions (Mondanlou & Freeman, 1982).

Although undulating patterns have been discussed under variability, the sinusoidal pattern is excluded from the definition of FHR variability (Parer, 1997). Undulating patterns are included here as they are evaluated when assessing baseline rate and variability.

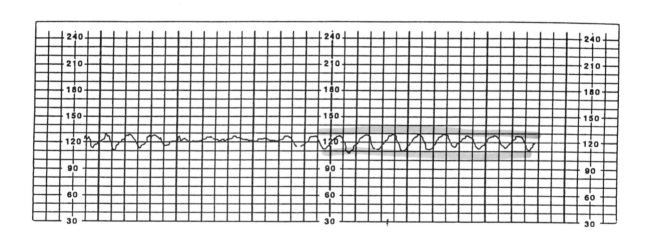

Figure 3-9. Example of sinusoidal pattern associated with feto-maternal hemorrhage.

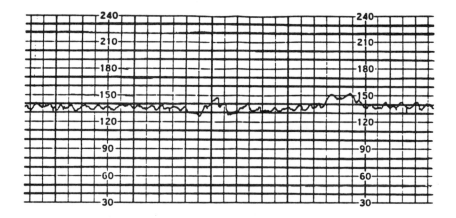

Figure 3-10. Example of an undulating, pseudosinusoidal pattern with normal periods of variability and reactivity.

Rhythm

Baseline	Fetal Heart Changes

Rate
    Normal
    Tachycardia
    Bradycardia
 	
Variability
    STV
    LTV
    Undulating
 	
RHYTHM
    REGULAR
    IRREGULAR	

Rhythm describes the regularity or irregularity of the baseline rate. It may be auscultated by the caregiver or recorded on the EFM tracing. It is annotated as regular or irregular.

Detection

The rhythm of the fetal heart may be initially noted by using most modes of FHM. As more sophisticated technology is employed to assess the fetal heart rhythm, more information can be obtained about the presence and nature of an irregular heartbeat. The irregular heart beat must be differentiated from possible artifact or electronic interference by verification using a technique such as auscultation, ultrasound scan, echocardiogram, or ECG. The presence of irregular heart beats can be verified by auscultation with a device allowing the practitioner to hear the heart sounds or with the fetal spiral electrode that detects cardiac electrical impulses. Information transmitted by ultrasound transducer or the spiral electrode mode often will illustrate a distinctive irregularity on the tracing, particularly if the logic button is disabled or the ECG switch is disabled. The latter method will graph an irregularity that must first be differentiated from possible artifact or electronic interference by verification with some other technique, such as auscultation, ultrasound scan, or echocardiogram. An ECG may be run simultaneously on monitors with this option. Most irregularities in the FHR display an organized pattern which distinguishes them from the chaotic appearance of artifact.

Types and characteristics of dysrhythmias

Two similar terms, arrhythmia and dysrhythmia, are used to describe irregular and abnormal rhythms of the fetal heart. A precise definition of arrhythmia, "without rhythm," describes the sporadic, irregular beats typical of the frequent fetal events heard or recorded on the tracing. This is often referred to as a sinus arrhythmia, as there is variability of R-to-R intervals, but with normal P waves occurring in a regular fashion preceding each QRS complex. Sinus arrhythmia is a normal fetal phenomenon and is categorized as a sinus node variant dysrhythmia (Cabaniss, 1993).

Dysrhythmia is defined as a fetal heart rhythm associated with a disordered impulse formation, impulse conduction, or a combination of both (Cabaniss, 1993). Most dysrhythmias are benign and require no intervention. However, what they do require from the professional is recognition, communication of the pattern to the appropriate personnel, and documentation. Most dysrhythmias will convert to a normal sinus rhythm shortly after birth; however, further assessment by a provider, via ultrasound or fetal echocardiogram, may be warranted depending on the dysrhythmia.

The terms arrhythmias and dysrhythmias are often used interchangeably by contemporary professionals. Selecting the term, arrhythmia or dysrhythmia, that more accurately describes irregular, sporadic events or an abnormal heart pattern may be correct but serves little practical purpose. The term dysrhythmia will be used in this brief overview of selected dysrhythmias. Dysrhythmias usually are categorized based upon the anatomical site of variant impulse formation, conduction, or a combination of both (Figure 3-11):

- Sinus node
- Supraventricular
- Ventricular
- Atrioventricular

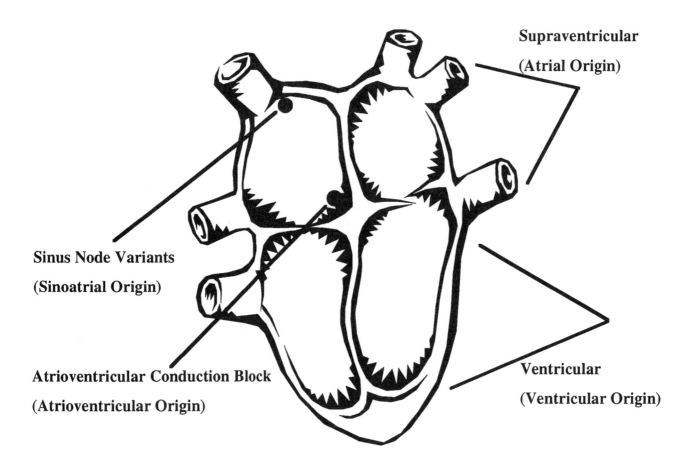

Figure 3-11. Types and characteristics of dysrhythmias

Sinus Node Variants   (SA node origin)

Most sinus node variants are patterns of baseline change discussed earlier in the chapter. The majority of these variants are common phenomena that usually have no effect on the well-being of the fetus, as there usually is no change in the true fetal ECG. Examples of sinus nodes variants include, but are not limited to (Figure 3-12)

- Sinus bradycardia.
- Sinus tachycardia

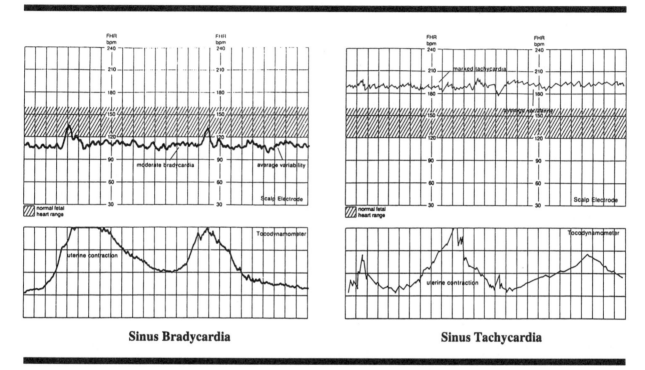

Sinus Bradycardia   **Sinus Tachycardia**

Figure 3-12. Examples of sinus node variants (Cabaniss, 1993)

93

Supraventricular Dysrhythmias   (Atrial origin)

Supraventricular dysrhythmias are often referred to as "premature beat" patterns and occur more commonly than "premature" ventricular dysrhythmic patterns. These dysrhythmias show actual changes in the fetal ECG. Atrial depolarization occurs prematurely and may result in an early P wave in relation to the QRS complex (Cabaniss, 1993). Typically these patterns are considered benign requiring no intervention other than observation. Regardless of the pattern, they tend to disappear in late labor, particularly during contractions, during variable decelerations, or soon after birth, and are usually not associated with any underlying cardiac disease (Cabaniss, 1993). These supraventricular dysrhythmia patterns can be combined with bigeminy, trigeminy, or a combination of both. Atrial bigeminy occurs when there is a premature atrial depolarization (contraction) every other beat. If the supraventricular dysrhythmic pattern occurs with bigeminy alone, the monitor tracing gives the appearance of two horizontal parallel lines (Cabaniss, 1993). Atrial trigeminy occurs when every third beat is a premature atrial depolarization (contraction). The trigeminal tracing will show vertical spikes with long upward strokes and short downward strokes (Figure 3-13). If the supraventricular dysrhythmic pattern occurs with bigeminy and trigeminy, the bigeminal pattern reveals a tracing that shows uninterrupted parallel vertical lines, often with the baseline obscured (Figure 3-13, Figure 3-14).

There are a few supraventricular dysrhythmia patterns of concern for the professional. One of those is supraventricular tachycardia (SVT) (Figure 3-15). SVT is a sustained rapid regular dysrhythmia of atrial origin in excess of 180-200 bpm. The monitoring tracing may show a loss of variability and half counting of the FHR. The undelivered or untreated fetus may develop cardiac failure and ischemic cerebral disease if SVT goes untreated. Treatment via pharmacologic cardioversion usually is successful in preventing or correcting fetal hydrops that is caused by cardiac failure, resultant of SVT. In short, SVT

- May be paroxysmal or continuous, characterized by a fixed R-R interval with P waves preceding each QRS complex as identified by ECG.

- May sometimes be pharmacologically cardioverted using digoxin, adenosine, verapamil, procainamide, quinidine, or propranolol via maternal route or percutaneous umbilical route.

- If prolonged or persistent, is a major risk of fetal heart failure or hydrops.

- May contribute to the newborn having an increased birth weight, heavier placenta, and diuresis of a few days' duration related to hydrops.

- May be associated with betamimetic therapy, such as ritodrine or terbutaline.

Another pattern of concern is SVT due to atrial flutter (Figure 3-15). With this pattern, the FHR is between 300 to 460 bpm, a rate too rapid for AV conduction. A 2:1 AV block then follows, with a slower ventricular rate present. The monitor tracing also may show half counting of the FHR. Pharmacologically, atrial flutter can be treated as SVT. However, echocardiography or ECG diagnosis in utero may alter prognosis and the plan of care.

Atrial fibrillation is another variation that may be associated with fetomaternal hemorrhage, neonatal Wolff-Parkinson-White syndrome, and cardiac structural abnormalities (Cabaniss, 1993).

- Antepartum diagnosis of this arrhythmia is rare.
- Atrial rates will vary from 300-460 bpm.
- Usually accompanied by a variable degree of AV block that will cause the ventricular rate to vary from 60-200 bpm.
- Electrocardiogram displays regularly recurring saw-toothed atrial activity instead of the normal P wave (atrial flutter) or low-amplitude irregular atrial activity with complexes of various sizes (atrial fibrillation).
- This arrhythmia rarely produces ascites or hydrops.
- Pharmacologic conversion may be successful.

Examples of supraventricular dysrhythmias (SVD) include, but are not limited to

- Premature atrial contraction (PAC) (Figure 3-13)
- Premature atrial contraction (PAC) with bigeminy (Figure 3-14)
- Premature atrial contraction (PAC) with trigeminy (Figure 3-13)
- Supraventricular tachycardia (SVT) (Figure 3-15)
- Atrial flutter (Figure 3-15)

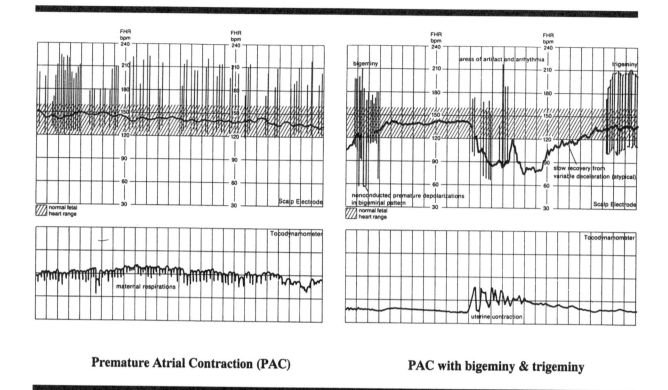

Premature Atrial Contraction (PAC)

PAC with bigeminy & trigeminy

Figure 3-13. Examples of supraventricular dysrhythmias (Cabaniss, 1993)

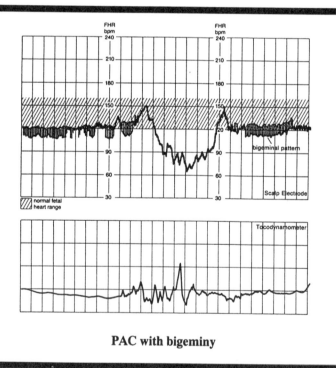

PAC with bigeminy

Figure 3-14. Another example of supraventricular dysrhythmias (Cabaniss, 1993)

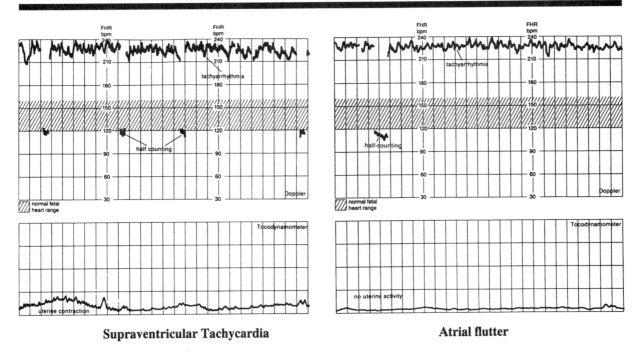

Supraventricular Tachycardia   **Atrial flutter**

Note: The tracings of these two dysrhythmias are indistinguishable. Further testing is necessary to distinguish the type of dysrhythmia present.

Figure 3-15. Additional examples of supraventricular dysrhythmias (Cabaniss, 1993)

<u>Ventricular Dysrhythmias</u>   (Ventricular origin)

Ventricular dysrhythmias are the result of premature electrical discharge below the AV junction (e.g., Bundle of HIS, Purkinje system, ventricle). Therefore, these patterns also are referred to as "premature beat" patterns. These ventricular dysrhythmias occur less frequently than supraventricular dysrhythmias and also show changes in the fetal ECG (e.g., absence of a P wave) (Cabaniss, 1993).

When these occur, the monitor tracing will show vertical spikes usually of equal distance above and below the normal FHR, usually resembling a "chimney." The monitor tracing also can appear as a vertical line downward and upward from the baseline, with the upward line appearing longer than the downward line. In this case, the unequal distance of the vertical line reflects the premature beat and compensatory pause of a premature ventricular contraction (PVC) (Figure 3-16). In the fetal spiral electrode (FSE) mode, as the electrical activity of the heart is displayed, a premature ventricular depolarization (or contraction) appears in the pattern described above. The ultrasound reflects the irregular motions of the heart wall or heart valve and displays this change. Usually these patterns tend to disappear in late labor, particularly during contractions or soon after birth. On occasion, pharmacologic therapy is used to correct the patterns, but is usually not warranted as the fetus seldom is jeopardized (Cabaniss, 1993).

Examples of ventricular dysrhythmias include, but are not limited to

- Premature Ventricular Contraction (PVC)
- PVC with bigeminy
- PVC with trigeminy

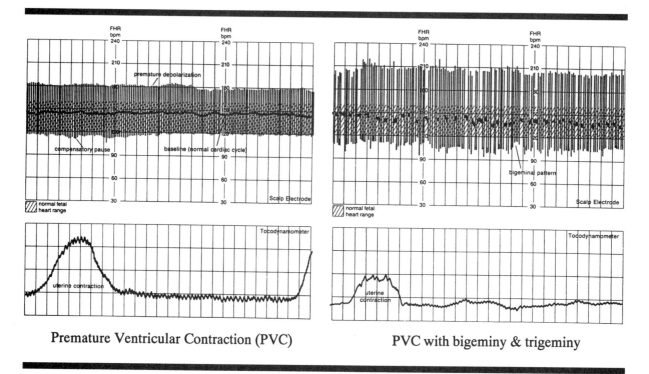

Premature Ventricular Contraction (PVC)   PVC with bigeminy & trigeminy

Figure 3-16. Examples of ventricular dysrhythmias (Cabaniss, 1993)

Regardless of whether the premature beat pattern is supraventricular or ventricular in nature, once the irregular beats are verified, their significance to the fetus is determined by evaluating the normal areas of the baseline for rate and variability, if present. When reactivity of the fetal heart (accelerations) is present along with LTV and STV, the significance of the dysrhythmic heartbeat is likely to be benign.

If the variability is nonreassuring/unfavorable (e.g., STV, LTV) and the fetal heart tracing demonstrates irregularity, the fetus needs further evaluation, such as an ultrasound, an echocardiogram, or ECG. It is important not to forget that under these circumstances, absence of variability may pertain more to neurologic defects or underlying defects than to the presence of fetal acidosis. In fact, interventions rarely are needed for fetal PVCs.

Key points regarding supraventricular and ventricular premature beats include the following:

- May originate from the supraventricular atrial or nodal areas or from the ventricular unifocal or multifocal areas.
- Rarely found in association with congenital cardiac defects.
- Significance usually is benign without the presence of other arrhythmias, murmurs, or detectable structural defects.
- Incidence is 3 - 8%.
- Caffeine, nicotine, and alcohol may be related.

Atrioventricular Block (AV node conduction defect)

First degree heart block is difficult to recognize in the fetus and has no known pathophysiology. Second degree heart block Mobitz type I (Wenckebach) is not seen in the fetus. Second degree heart block Mobitz type II is difficult to diagnosis in the fetus because the atrial and ventricular rates may appear as the same rate. Third degree heart block, or complete heart block in the fetus is associated with maternal collagen vascular disease which produces fetal cardiac tissue damage (Figure 3-17). Fetal hydrops developing from an immune mechanism responds to maternally administered steroid therapy. Congenital complete AV block is associated with a 30-50% risk of congenital cardiac malformations. It also has been associated with fetal cytomegalovirus infection. Key points to be considered are

- First degree heart block does appear in the fetus.
- Second-degree (AV) heart block is associated with rapid atrial rates due to SVT, atrial flutter, or atrial fibrillation. The block represents failure of some of the atrial impulses to be conducted.
- Third-degree block or complete AV block represents complete absence of conduction of P waves. The following facts are associated with this dysrhythmia:
  -- Incidence is 1 per 20,000 live births.
  -- FHR monitoring shows a 50-70 bpm ventricular rate unless the external doppler is placed over the fetal atria. A rapid rate will then appear.
  -- 50-65% of mothers whose fetuses exhibit complete AV block will have laboratory or clinical evidence of connective tissue disease, such as systemic lupus erythematosus (SLE).

Examples Atrioventricular Block (AV Block) include, but are not limited to

- Second-degree AV block
- Third-degree AV block (Figure 3-17)

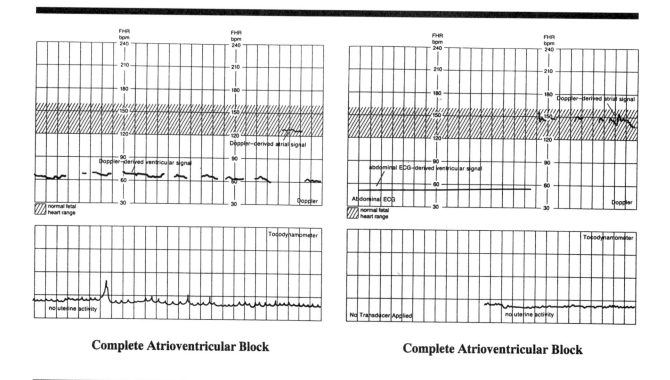

Figure 3-17. Two examples of complete atrioventricular block (third degree heart block) (Cabaniss, 1993)

Periodic Patterns

As the fetal heart accelerates and decelerates away from the baseline rate in direct relation to uterine contractions, the response is classified as a periodic pattern or a periodic change. Based upon the appearance of the pattern, it may receive a descriptive label and a presumed underlying physiology. For example, alterations of fetal blood flow via the umbilical cord or alterations of the uteroplacental unit are presumed based upon their characteristic pattern appearances.

Periodic Accelerations

Baseline	Fetal Heart Changes

Rate
  Normal
  Tachycardia
  Bradycardia
 	
Variability
  STV
  LTV
  Undulating
 	
Rhythm
  Regular
  Irregular
	Periodic
	
	ACCELERATIONS

Periodic Acceleration Physiology

Periodic accelerations are those which occur with contractions. There are currently several theories that explain the etiology. One explanation is that a mild compression of the umbilical cord with the contraction may occlude only the umbilical vein. The decrease in blood flow to the fetus decreases systemic blood pressure, which triggers a compensatory acceleration of the FHR. A second explanation is direct sympathetic stimulation of the fetus. Some hypothesize that fundal pressure exerted on the vertex of a breech presentation also may elicit a sympathetic response and acceleration. A third reason for these accelerations may be fetal movement during contractions.

Periodic Acceleration Characteristics

- May occur simultaneously with the uterine contraction.
- May be smoother in configuration.
- May be biphasic or triphasic.
- Often forerunners of a variable deceleration pattern.

Periodic Acceleration Assessment

- Assess the acceleration for amplitude, duration, and shape.
- Note the presence or absence of baseline variability.
- Remember that double-peaked accelerations have been associated with minor cord compression.

Variable Decelerations

Baseline	Fetal Heart Changes
Rate 　　Normal 　　Tachycardia 　　Bradycardia Variability 　　STV 　　LTV 　　Undulating Rhythm 　　Regular 　　Irregular	Periodic Accelerations **DECELERATIONS** 　　**VARIABLE**

Variable decelerations are abrupt decelerations of the FHR in response to cord compression. The umbilical vessels can be partially compressed so that the thinner walled umbilical vein is compressed first. This compression slows the blood flowing toward the fetus, decreases cardiac output and, hence, causes the blood pressure to fall. The fetus compensates for this change by raising the heart rate to increase cardiac output. As the umbilical compression continues to develop, compresses the artery and occludes the arterial flow moving away from the fetus, the blood pressure escalates and triggers the baroreceptor response. These hemodynamic changes are presumed to trigger the vagal response resulting in an abrupt drop in FHR.

Variable Deceleration Physiology

- Caused by decreased umbilical cord perfusion, usually occurring when the umbilical cord is compressed; may lead to hypoxemia hypercarbic responses.

- Compressing the umbilical cord stimulates a baroreceptor response. The baroreceptor response originates in the carotid bodies and aortic arch and is transmitted to the midbrain and then to the PSNS.

- Partial cord compression causes umbilical vein compression first, followed by umbilical arterial compression. Umbilical vein compression is thought to stimulate the acceleration phases that may precede or follow variable decelerations. The umbilical arterial compression leads to the actual deceleration phase of the variable.

- Parasympathetic responses slow the heart rate via the sinus node in response to the fetal systemic blood pressure, resulting in decreased blood pressure.

- The variable deceleration pattern may include an acceleration phase that precedes or follows the deceleration. This increase in the FHR is a component of the variable deceleration pattern. The acceleration component is a physiologic compensatory response to hypoxemia (oxygen deprivation). Shoulders are not associated with poor outcome (Schifrin & Clement, 1990).

- The term "shoulder" describes a compensatory acceleration that may precede or follow the deceleration, with an increase in rate generally less than 20 bpm, and lasting less than 20 seconds. When short term variability is present, the pattern is reassuring.

- The term "overshoot" or "rebound overshoot" describes a compensatory acceleration that only follows the deceleration, with an increase in rate generally greater than 20 bpm and lasting more than 20 seconds. When overshoots are repetitive and short term variability is absent, the pattern is nonreassuring.

- Other descriptions of the acceleration component of the variable deceleration pattern include "primary and secondary acceleratory phases of the deceleration pattern" (Murray, 1996, p. 261) and "variable accelerations" (Afriat, 1996, p. 208; Schifrin & Clement, 1990).

Variable Deceleration Characteristics

- The most common periodic deceleration pattern.
- The timing of the deceleration may vary in its onset and offset.
- Shape, depth, and duration vary (Figure 3-19).
- Usually abrupt and decelerate quickly (onset to nadir uaually < 30 seconds).
- May resemble or be in combination with other pattern types.
- May have accelerations before or after the deceleration (Figure 3-18).
  -- shoulders
  -- overshoots

- Changing the maternal position may alter its shape, depth, and duration to improve or worsen the pattern.

- Shape may be U, V, or W, or may mimic other patterns. W-shape is more common when the umbilical cord is long or the cord is wrapped around the fetal body (Welt, 1984).

- Often referred to as "variables."

The frequency and significance of the various features of variable decelerations have been described by Krebs, Petres, & Dunn (1983). Atypical features were identified as characteristics more commonly associated with hypoxemia. The listing of atypical features which follows, indicates the significance and frequency of each feature. Note that the most significant feature indicating fetal hypoxemia, loss of variability, is fortunately one of the least frequently occurring (Table 3-1).

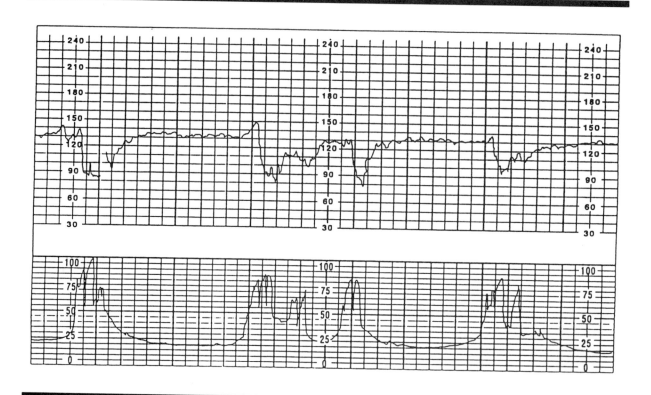

Figure 3-18. Example of variable decelerations with and without "shoulders."

Atypical Features of Variable Decelerations

<u>Significance</u>	<u>Frequency</u>
1st Loss of variability	6th
2nd Loss of secondary acceleration only if accompanied by #1	3rd
3rd Biphasic deceleration	5th
4th Prolonged secondary acceleration	4th
5th Slow return to baseline	2nd
6th Continuation of baseline at lower level	7th
7th Loss of initial acceleration	1st

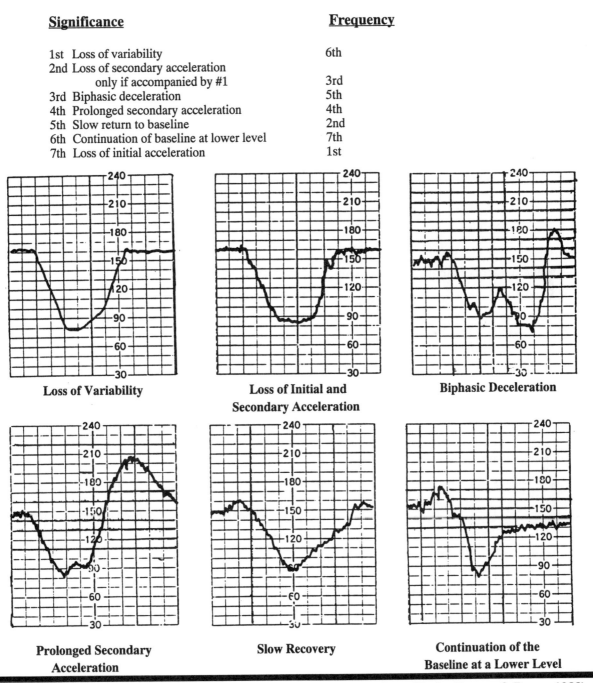

Table 3-1. Atypical Features of variable decelerations (Adapted from Krebs, Petres, & Dunn, 1983)

Additional research (ACOG, 1995b; Freeman et al., 1991) has supported these findings and further identifies variable decelerations as reassuring and nonreassuring.

Reassuring Variable Deceleration Characteristics

- Lasting no more than 30 - 45 seconds.
- Rapid return to baseline.
- Accompanied by normal baseline rate and variability.
  (Freeman et al., 1991)

Nonreassuring Variable Deceleration Characteristics

- Prolonged return to baseline.
- Presence of overshoots.
- Rising baseline.
- Absence or loss of STV and/or LTV.
- Development of tachycardia (Freeman et al., 1991).
- Persistent to < 70 bpm and > 60 seconds (ACOG, 1995b).

Variable Deceleration Etiology

- Short umbilical cord.
- Nuchal cord.
- Body entanglement of umbilical cord.
- Occult or obvious prolapse of umbilical cord.
- Second stage of labor/descent of fetus.
- Decreased amniotic fluid.
- Other umbilical cord abnormalities.
  -- knot in cord
  -- decreased Wharton's Jelly

Variable Deceleration Assessment

- Depth and duration of nadir.
- The deceleration from onset to nadir is typically 30 seconds or less.
- Duration of recovery time.
- Variability in the subsequent baseline and during the decelerations, nadir, and recovery.
- Trend in baseline rate (higher, lower).
- Presence of atypical features of variable decelerations as described by Krebs et al. (1983).

106

- Presence of shoulders versus overshoots.
- Stage and progress of labor.
  -- Second-stage variables are common and considered benign when adequate variability is present

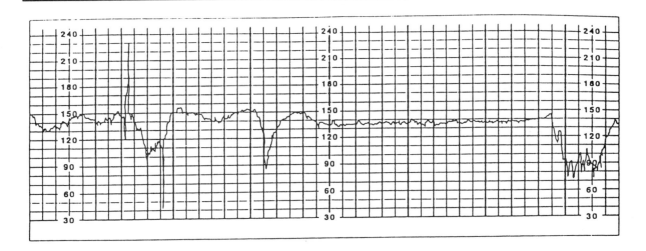

Figure 3-19. Examples of variable decelerations. Exhibits a variety of possible shapes including U, V, and W.

Late Decelerations

Baseline	Fetal Heart Changes
Rate 　Normal 　Tachycardia 　Bradycardia Variability 　STV 　LTV 　Undulating Rhythm 　Regular 　Irregular	Periodic Accelerations **DECELERATIONS** 　Variable 　**LATE**

Late decelerations must have two characteristics, timing and shape, to be called late decelerations. To understand the late timing of this pattern, one must review the exchange of oxygen between the maternal and fetal circulation. When the uteroplacental exchange of blood actually occurs, its imminent effect on the fetus cannot be evaluated. The late response is due to the time it takes for uteroplacental blood flow to reach the fetal heart and brain. The fetal brain and heart then will respond to the amount of blood and oxygen received. This event is referred to as lag time.

A pattern of persistent late decelerations requires prompt attention and intervention. Late decelerations may be precipitated by the following physiologic events: altered maternal blood flow to the placenta, reduced maternal arterial oxygen saturation, or placental changes altering maternal-fetal gas exchange.

Late Deceleration Physiology

- Diminished uterine blood flow with contraction.
- Critical reduction of pO_2 following peak of contraction.
- Reflex slowing (vagal) of heart rate.
- Hypoxic slowing (local) of heart rate.

Late Deceleration Characteristics

- The shape of the decelerations is uniform, symmetrical, and smooth, and often reflects the intensity of the contraction.
- The deceleration usually begins 20-30 seconds after the onset of the contraction, usually at or after the peak of the contraction.
- The deceleration typically requires greater than 30 seconds from beginning to nadir.
- The deceleration returns to baseline after the contraction ends.
- The nadir (bottom) of the deceleration is offset or after the acme (peak) of the contraction.
- The nadir commonly decreases 5-30 bpm and rarely 30-40 bpm below the baseline (may be small or "subtle" in appearance but not in significance).
- The baseline rate may be increasing with repetitive late decelerations.
- The variability may be average, decreased, or absent.
- The decelerations are repetitive.

    (Hon, 1975; Freeman et al., 1991; Parer, 1989, 1997; Petrie, 1991)

Late Deceleration Etiologic Factors

- Maternal factors that may decrease uteroplacental circulation.
    -- Hypotension*
        --- supine position*
        --- maternal trauma or blood loss*
        --- regional anesthesia*

-- Hypertension

--- pregnancy-induced or chronic hypertension

--- medications (e.g., illicit drugs, such as cocaine and amphetamines)

-- Uterine hyperstimulation or hypertonus with or without oxytocin or prostaglandin administration

- Physiologic conditions that may be associated with decreased maternal arterial hemoglobin/oxygen saturation.

-- hyperventilation*

-- hypoventilation *

-- cardiopulmonary disease

- Placental changes that may affect uteroplacental gas exchange.

-- postmaturity

-- premature aging, including calcification, necrosis

-- old and new abruptio sites

-- placenta previa

-- placental malformation

- Increased association with other high-risk conditions of pregnancy.

-- chronic maternal diseases, such as diabetes and collagen disease

-- maternal smoking

-- poor maternal nutrition

-- multiple gestation

-- anemia

Late Deceleration Assessment

- Depth, duration, and timing in relation to contractions.
- Uniformity in shape.
- Persistence of pattern.
- Variability during the subsequent baseline.
- Changes in baseline (e.g., rise) and loss of baseline variability.
- Effectiveness of interventions.

* May be associated with <u>reflex late decelerations,</u> which are more likely to be reversed with interventions (Parer, 1989; Petrie, 1991).

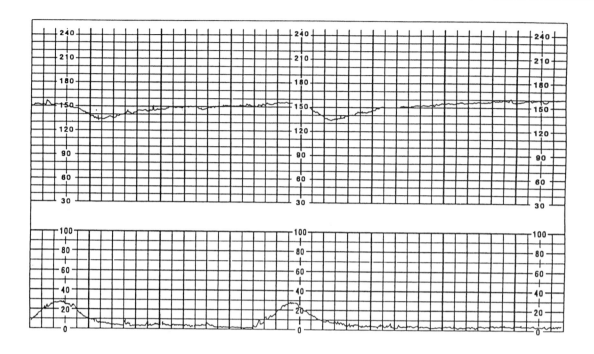

Figure 3-20. Example of late decelerations with absent STV & decreased LTV.

Early Decelerations

Baseline	Fetal Heart Changes

Rate
    Normal
    Tachycardia
    Bradycardia
 	
Variability
    STV
    LTV
    Undulating
 	
Rhythm
    Regular
    Irregular
	Periodic
	———————————
	Accelerations
	DECELERATIONS
	    Variable
	    Late
	    EARLY

An early deceleration is a gradual decrease in the FHR associated with compression of the fetal head during uterine contractions. Head compression is thought to precipitate a reflex vagal response. Early decelerations are thought to be benign.

Early Deceleration Physiology

- Occurs more frequently in primigravidas.
- Occurs more often during early active labor, usually 4-7 cm.
- Higher association with cephalopelvic disproportion, unengaged presenting part in early labor, or persistent occipitut posterior presentation.
- Reflex vagal response.
- The mechanism is not associated with level of oxygenation.

Early Deceleration Characteristics

- The deceleration mirrors and occurs simultaneously with the contraction (Figure 3-21).
- The shape is uniform.
- Nadir usually is reached at the same time as peak of uterine contraction.

  (ACOG, 1995b; Hon, 1975; Freeman et al., 1991; Parer, 1989)

Early Deceleration Assessments

- Timing of pattern to rule out late deceleration pattern.
- Maternal position changes do not usually alter pattern.
- Baseline variability during the subsequent baseline is present.
- Characteristics of early decelerations listed previously.

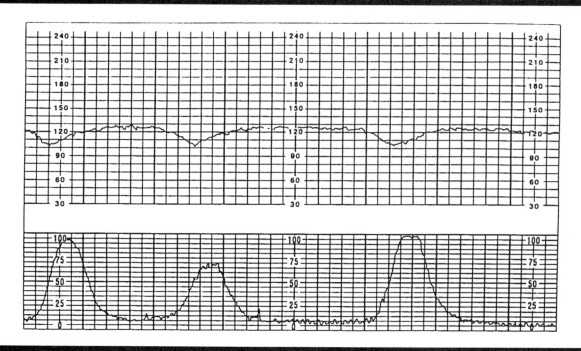

Figure 3-21. Example of early decelerations in a pattern with active labor and cephalopelvic disproportion.

Combined Deceleration Patterns

Baseline	Fetal Heart Changes

Rate
    Normal
    Tachycardia
    Bradycardia
 	
Variability
    STV
    LTV
    Undulating
 	
Rhythm
    Regular
    Irregular
	Periodic
	———————————————
	Accelerations
	DECELERATIONS
	    Variable
	    Late
	    Early
	    COMBINED DECELERATION PATTERNS

Fetal monitoring instruction defines each pattern type separately, often omitting the fact that various types of patterns may appear consecutively or simultaneously. The terminology used, such as late, variable, and early deceleration, suggests that only a single deceleration pattern may exist for a given patient. Considering the physiology of deceleration patterns and the complexity of pregnancy, it is possible to have patterns that cannot be classified as early, late, or variable deceleration patterns. These patterns may result when more than one mechanism causes a combination of "single" deceleration patterns and contain characteristics of both of the "single" patterns in regard to shape and timing. However, most patterns are not combined.

Assessment/interpretation of single deceleration patterns can be difficult enough without adding components of other patterns. Yet, assessment/interpretation of combined deceleration patterns is simplified by looking at the main factors used when assessing/interpreting any deceleration: shape and timing, and variability.

Two cases will be used to illustrate the complex physiology. In the first case, a fetus may be experiencing cord compression and intrauterine growth restriction, coupled with maternal pre-eclampsia. In this case, the fetus has a placenta that is not capable of oxygenating the fetus related to uteroplacental insufficiency. In addition, available oxygen for the fetus is decreased related to decreased umbilical circulation. Therefore, uteroplacental insufficiency is coupled with cord compression. Having both physiologic mechanisms of late and variable decelerations occurring at the same time may result in a fetal heart deceleration pattern with "late" timing and "variable" shape (Figure 3-22).

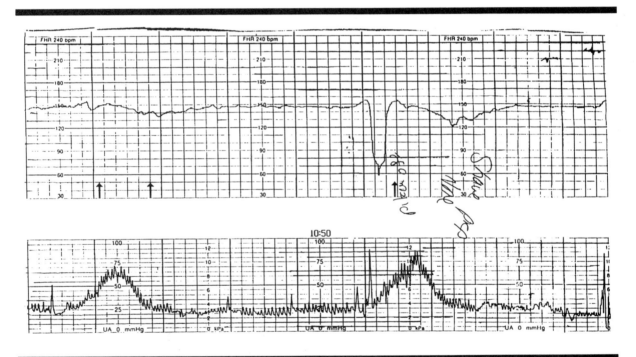

Figure 3-22. Example of combination deceleration pattern of variable and late decelerations

In a second case, a primiparous patient pushing with a fetus experiencing cord compression may also result in more than one distinct deceleration pattern occuring. Pushing may be associated with head compression and a reflex vagal response associated with alterations in cerebral blood flow patterns. Both physiologic mechanisms of early and variable decelerations may occur at the same time, causing the fetal heart deceleration to demonstrate "early" timing and "variable" shape (Figure 3-23).

113

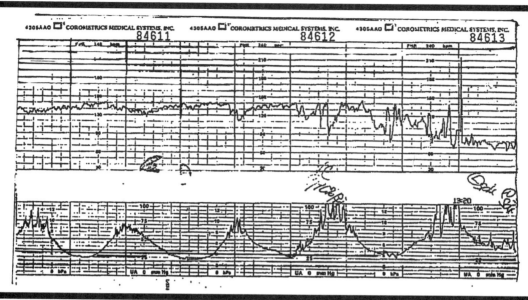

Figure 3-23. Example of combination deceleration pattern of variable and early decelerations

What terminology is used to describe patterns that do not resemble classic descriptions of early, late, or variable decelerations? The literature is scattered with phrases such as, "late variables" (Cabaniss, 1993), "early variables" (Cabaniss, 1993), and "variables with late components" (Eden, 1989). Regardless of what these patterns are referred to as, it is important to recognize that combined deceleration patterns can exist based on the underlying physiology. Recognizing that these patterns exist is important, yet what is most important is to remember that the FHR baseline and variability should always be assessed in addition to the deceleration pattern recovery time observed. Presence of or return to a normal FHR baseline, average LTV, and present STV, provides some reassurance that the fetus is tolerating the deceleration pattern. Presence of accelerations indicates a fetus is well oxygenated with an intact nervous system. Continued assessment of all FHR parameters is indicated as with any single deceleration pattern. Interventions will be based on the entire individual clinical picture. Documentation of such tracings involves describing, a) what is seen with regard to shape and timing, b) what interventions were done, and c) the outcome of the interventions. For additional information about interventions, see Chapter 4.

Nonperiodic Patterns

Decelerations and accelerations may appear unassociated with uterine contractions. When this transpires, the event or pattern is described as nonperiodic. Some authors (Afriat, 1989; Murray, 1996) refer to these patterns as "spontaneous changes/patterns." Accelerations are the most common nonperiodic FHR event (Figure 3-24).

Nonperiodic Accelerations

Baseline	Fetal Heart Changes	
Rate		
Normal	Periodic	**NONPERIODIC**
Tachycardia		
Bradycardia	Accelerations	**ACCELERATIONS**
	Decelerations	
Variability	Variable	
STV	Late	
LTV	Early	
Undulating	Combined deceleration	
	patterns	
Rhythm		
Regular		
Irregular		

Nonperiodic Acceleration Physiology

- Occurs in response to environmental stimuli or fetal activity.
- A reassuring event indicating an intact, oxygenated sympathetic innervation.
- Associated with a nonacidotic, oxygenated, active fetus.
- Younger fetuses (< 28 weeks of gestation) may demonstrate accelerations.

Nonperiodic Acceleration Characteristics

- A reassuring or favorable acceleration increases at least 15 beats above the baseline, and the acceleration spans at least 15 seconds.
- The shape of the acceleration is often peaked or abrupt.

Nonperiodic Acceleration Assessment

- Assess the acceleration for amplitude, duration, and shape.
- Note the presence or absence of baseline variability.

- Note fetal movement.
- Note that once accelerations are demonstrated, the fetus should be able to maintain this ability to accelerate its heart rate.

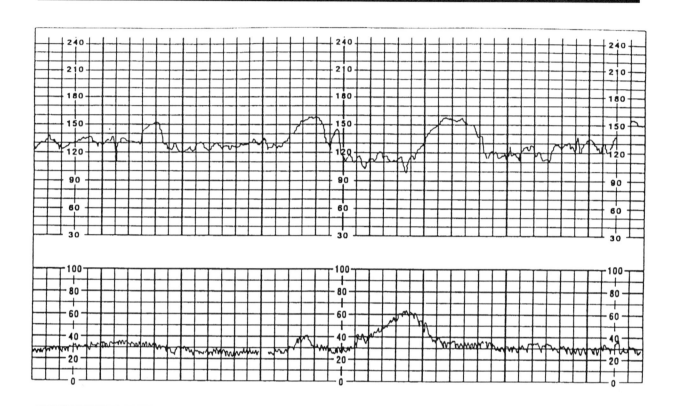

Figure 3-24. Example of nonperiodic accelerations

Nonperiodic Variable Decelerations

Baseline	Fetal Heart Changes	

Rate
    Normal
    Tachycardia
    Bradycardia
 	
Variability
    STV
    LTV
    Undulating
 	
Rhythm
    Regular
    Irregular
	Periodic — **NONPERIODIC**
	
	Accelerations
	Decelerations
	    Variable
	    Late
	    Early
	    Combined deceleration
	        patterns
		Accelerations
		DECELERATIONS
		VARIABLE

Nonperiodic variable decelerations may occur prior to labor indicating cord compression just as the periodic variable decelerations do. According to antepartum nonstress testing criteria, variable decelerations that decrease 15 bpm or more with a duration of at least 15 seconds should receive further evaluation. In such cases, either oligohydramnios or umbilical cord entanglement may be present. Cases exist in which variable decelerations have been documented in conjunction with fetal movement. The attending practitioner should evaluate the frequency and severity of the decelerations, gestation, and overall prenatal status for each pregnancy (ACOG, 1995b) (Figure 3-25).

Nonperiodic Variable Deceleration Physiology

- Mechanism of cord compression is the same as with periodic variable decelerations.
- May be associated with decreased amniotic fluid volume (oligohydramnios) or cord entanglement.
- More often associated with fetal movement and cord entanglement.

Nonperiodic Variable Deceleration Characteristics

- Resembles characteristics of periodic decelerations.
- May be of shorter duration and of less depth than periodic variables, but may be more significant depending upon maternal-fetal history.

Nonperiodic Variable Deceleration Etiology

- Similar to periodic decelerations.

- May be found with chronic conditions or changes associated with decreased amniotic fluid (e.g., postmaturity).

Nonperiodic Variable Deceleration Assessment

- Refer to assessment of periodic variable deceleration beginning on page 105.

- Assess significant maternal-fetal historical and physical data (e.g., gestational age, biophysical profile).

- Assess variability in the subsequent baseline (taking gestational age into consideration).

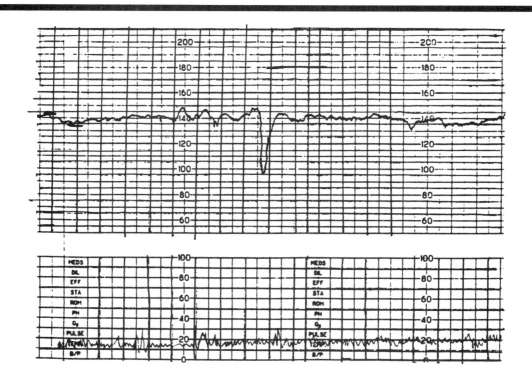

Figure 3-25. Example of nonperiodic variable deceleration

Nonperiodic Prolonged Deceleration

Baseline	Fetal Heart Changes	
Rate		
Normal	Periodic	**NONPERIODIC**
Tachycardia		
Bradycardia	Accelerations	Accelerations
	Decelerations	**DECELERATIONS**
Variability	Variable	Variable
STV	Late	**PROLONGED**
LTV	Early	
Undulating	Combined deceleration	
	patterns	
Rhythm		
Regular		
Irregular		

Prolonged decelerations are decelerations of the FHR lasting greater than or equal to two minutes, but less than or equal to 10 minutes (Figure 3-26). Prolonged decelerations are considered nonperiodic as they occur in response to stimuli (possibly a contraction) but are generally not repetitious. The most important thing with prolonged decelerations is to look for an identifiable cause and correct the problem, if possible, to prevent further prolonged decelerations. Although prolonged decelerations may appear dramatic, most can be modified with such simple interventions as position change.

Prolonged decelerations and sudden bradycardias may be activated when profound changes occur in the fetal environment, such as extensive abruptio placentae, uterine hypertonus or hyperstimulus drug reactions, terminal fetal conditions, maternal death, and cord accidents. These decelerations also may occur in response to other changes, such as hypotension associated with drug responses (e.g., sympathetic blockade with anesthesia) or occasionally vagal stimulation with a vaginal examination or the Valsalva maneuver (Afriat, 1996; Tucker, 1996). Less frequent causes of prolonged decelerations include cord impingement (due to short cord, true knot in the cord, or umbilical cord thrombosis), cord prolapse, uterine rupture, maternal seizures, status asthmaticus, or maternal cardiorespiratory collapse (Cabaniss, 1993; Tucker, 1996). Prolonged decelerations also may appear when the cord is compressed for a substantial time, perhaps following maternal position change or fetal movement. The etiology in such situations corresponds to that of a variable deceleration.

Prolonged Deceleration Physiology

- Dependent on the precipitating cause.
- Associated with baroreceptors, chemoreceptors, autonomic nervous system, and CNS responses to profound changes in fetal environment.

Prolonged Deceleration Characteristics

- Duration of 2 or more minutes, but usually less than 10 minutes.
- Note: A rebound response may be associated with prolonged decelerations. Transient fetal tachycardia and loss of variability may be associated with profound episodes (ACOG, 1995b).

Prolonged Deceleration Possible Etiology

- Umbilical cord compression
  - -- Prolonged cord compression
  - -- Short cord
  - -- Cord accidents
  - -- Oligohydramnios with decreased Wharton's jelly
- Hypertonic uterine activity
  - -- Abruptio placentae
  - -- Maternal uterine hypertonus
  - -- Medications (e.g., oxytocin)
- Altered maternal condition
  - -- Hypotension
  - -- Maternal position
  - -- Side effect of medication (e.g., analgesia or anesthesia)
  - -- Convulsions
  - -- Respiratory arrest
  - -- Sustained maternal Valsalva maneuvers
  - -- Hypoxia
- Procedures
  - -- Vaginal examination
  - -- Fetal blood sampling
  - -- Application of internal fetal monitor
- Rapid fetal descent

Prolonged Deceleration Assessment

- Duration
- Depth
- Return to baseline
- Baseline FHR variability after insult
- Possible causes
- Response to interventions

The degree to which such decelerations are nonreassuring depends on their depth and duration, loss of variability, response of fetus during recovery, and, most importantly, the frequency and progression of recurrence (ACOG, 1995b). Prolonged hypoxia also is a factor in the etiology of prolonged decelerations. The impact of uterine activity has been cited in several instances as a factor in fetal heart decelerations and intrauterine events. The intrapartum uterine activity not only alters blood flow to the fetus, but influences the duration of labor and the repeated intrapartum physiologic stresses. It is worthwhile to consider, briefly, factors that affect uterine activity.

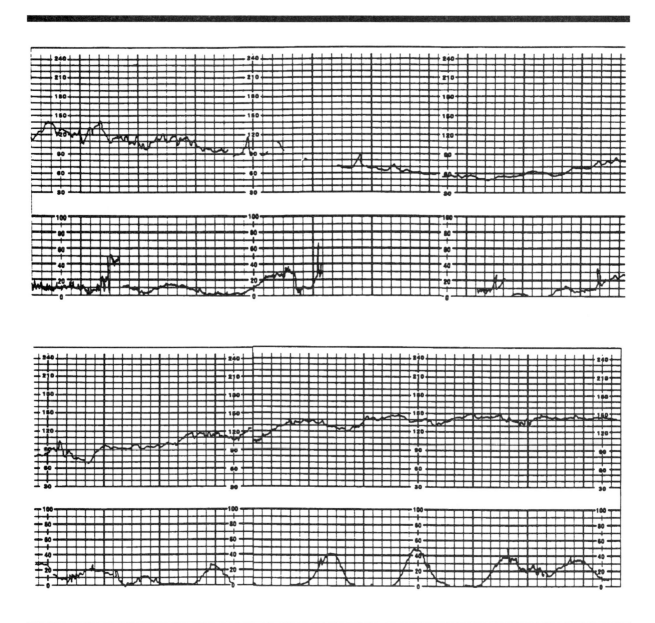

Figure 3-26. Example of nonperiodic prolonged deceleration

Summary of Fetal Heart Baseline Rate and Changes

Baseline	Fetal Heart Changes	
Rate		
Normal	Periodic	Nonperiodic
Tachycardia		
Bradycardia	Accelerations	Accelerations
	Decelerations	Decelerations
Variability	Variable	Variable
STV	Late	Prolonged
LTV	Early	
Undulating	Combined deceleration	
	patterns	
Rhythm		
Regular		
Irregular		

Uterine Activity

Effective labor occurs when rhythmic uterine contractions of adequate frequency, intensity, and duration result in cervical effacement and dilatation with descent of the presenting part.

Factors Affecting Labor

Factors affecting labor constitute those that are fixed and cannot be changed, as well as those that are dynamic or changeable. Those that cannot be changed are maternal age, parity, relative health status, pelvic size and shape, fetal size, presentation (that did not convert with external version), and gestational age. Factors that may be changed to some degree are hydration, maternal psychological status and anxiety, intensity and duration of contractions, maternal position, pushing, drugs, and medication.

Fetal situations contributing to labor dystocia may include a problem with size, position, or anatomy. Abnormal labor patterns due to these fetal problems may persist until the problems are corrected with rotation or delivery (Friedman, 1978; Perkins, 1987).

Hydration

Hydration often is overlooked as an influence on labor because the onset of dehydration is gradual. Maternal fluid loss occurs with perspiration, rapid and heavy breathing, vomiting, and body maintenance needs. This situation is compounded when fluid intake prior to admission to labor and delivery is poor, creating the potential for fluid volume deficit. The hydrated patient also responds to induction or augmentation better than a dehydrated patient. Dehydrated patients usually respond well to early treatment with intravenous hydration of an isotonic, nondextrose electrolyte solution. An infusion may improve labor progress, as well as endurance, thereby avoiding or lessening the need for augmentation.

122

Caution must be taken to avoid overloading the patient with high dextrose or hypotonic intravenous fluids. Infusion overloads of > 5% dextrose or hypotonic solutions can lead to glycosuria, osmotic diuresis, and/or maternal and neonatal hyponatremia (Grylack, Chu, & Scanlog, 1984; Morton, Jackson, & Gillmer, 1985; Singhi & Chookang, 1984).

Oral hydration also can be used as a means to hydrate a patient. As controversial as this issue can be, there is neither evidence to show benefit to withholding oral fluids, nor evidence of risk in allowing oral fluids during labor. However, it is recommended that oral hydration be restricted to non-particulate fluids (Elkington, 1991).

<u>Maternal Anxiety</u>

Maternal anxiety can influence the labor progress. Anxiety or fear stimulates the adrenal glands to secrete catecholamines (adrenaline, epinephrine, norepinephrine, etc.) that bind with uterine B receptors. This action leads to ineffective uterine activity, which increases the risk of dysfunctional labor. It also can increase the duration of the first stage of labor, and decrease Montevideo units (Arnold-Aldea & Parer, 1990; Lederman, Lederman, Work, & McCann, 1978; Murray, 1996; Simpkin, 1986). When anxiety is present, uterine contractions also can be described as increased in frequency and tachysystole, but decreased in strength and duration (Fenwick & Simpkin, 1987; Friedman, 1978, 1989; Lederman, Lederman, Work, & McCann, 1985).

Maternal anxiety can also influence the fetal heart rate. The adrenaline produced when anxiety is present dilates other vessels in the body. This generalized dilation then decreases uterine blood flow and can result in bradycardia (Petrie, 1986; Simpkin, 1986). Oxygen delivery to the fetus decreases, which may decrease fetal oxygen and pH levels and increase fetal CO_2 levels. As a result, fetal blood pressure falls, causing decelerations and/or bradycardia (Arnold-Aldea & Parer, 1990; Murray, 1996; Myers, 1975). Researchers have noted that when pregnant monkeys become frightened, the fetus demonstrates bradycardia.

Considering this physiologic response to maternal anxiety, it is easy to see the importance of using anxiety-relieving measures in the laboring patient to include coaching support. The assistance, support, coaching presence, and information given by caregivers apparently has a physiologic influence on labor (Bowes, 1989). For example, when intrapartum women use information they have learned in prenatal classes, a shorter average labor results (approximately 2-3 hours less) (Friedman, 1978).

<u>Intensity and Duration of Labor</u>

Dystocia (subnormal or abnormal uterine contractions) requires the assessment of the power, passenger, and pelvis for correctable causes. Although a wide range of power has been found in "adequate labor" (uterine contractions every 2-4.5 minutes, with 25-75 mm Hg, and 95-395 Montevideo units), direct monitoring is recommended for assessing the status of labor when a) "the latent phase of labor has been completed with the cervix dilated 4 cm or more or b) a uterine contraction pattern of ≥ 200 Montevideo units in a 10-minute period has been present for 2 hours without cervical change" (ACOG, 1995). Montevideo units are derived by subtracting the resting tone from the peak pressure in mm Hg for each uterine contraction that occurs in a 10-minute period. The pressures obtained are then added together for the total number of Montevideo units in that 10-minute period. If the baseline resting tone is within normal limits for the type of IUPC used, the baseline pressure may be subtracted from peak pressure values. It is appropriate to describe the uterine contractions and the baseline tonus in actual millimeters of mercury (mm Hg) when communicating these events.

The literature suggests that time (2-3 hours) be used to correct an abnormal labor in the first stage, as well as the length of the second stage of labor. As long as progress in descent (not molding/caput) is noted, and fetal surveillance demonstrates the absence of unfavorable or nonreassuring patterns, the duration of the second stage of labor is unrelated to outcome. Waiting may be the most appropriate decision (Cohen, Acker, & Freidman, 1989; Schifrin & Cohen, 1989).

Maternal Position and Pushing

Assessment in the second stage of labor may include anesthesia, analgesia, maternal pushing effort, maternal position that enhances uterine blood flow and uterine activity, and pain relief. The etiology of dystocia may be related to abnormalities of the uterine myofibrils, nerve innervation, structural abnormalities, excessive analgesia, maternal fatigue, or hormonal/enzyme function (ACOG, 1995a; Garfield, 1987; Huszar & Roberts, 1982; May & Mahlmeister, 1994). Dysfunctional contractions may be physiologically described as subnormal (or hypotonic), hypertonic, or abnormal. These dysfunctional contractions can be more frequent in occurrence and less effective. During induction, frequency also may be mistaken for effectiveness, especially if the intensity and duration of contractions are not assessed (ACOG, 1995a). The uterus may be unable to contract effectively as seen by hypotonus, hypertonus, or abnormal tracings. It is imperative to define an abnormal contraction pattern so that appropriate therapy may be instituted. Supine positioning and the consequential reduction in uterine blood flow can cause uterine contractions to become more frequent, less intense, and therefore less effective (Abitbol, 1985; Carlson, Diehl, Sachtleben-Murray, McRae, Fenwick, & Friedman, 1986; Fenwick & Simpkin, 1987).

Drugs and Medications

Agents that alter uterine contractions and have potential fetal effects include pitocin, prostaglandin, magnesium sulfate, betasympathomimetics, antiprostaglandins (indomethacin), and illicit drugs (cocaine, amphetamine) (Baxi & Petrie, 1987). Oxytocin administered for induction or augmentation necessitates close evaluation or monitoring because individual sensitivity and clearance rates vary. ACOG/AWHONN guidelines discuss administration of Pitocin and induction/augmentation of labor in detail (ACOG, 1991). Prostaglandin administration for ripening the cervix or induction also necessitates close observation, especially during the first 4 hours following administration, due to individual sensitivity and response (ACOG, 1991; AWHONN, 1993).

Betasympathomimetics, prostaglandin synthetase inhibitors (PGSI), magnesium sulfate, and calcium channel blockers frequently are used to treat preterm labor. Close assessment and documentation of the uterine pattern and fetal response are essential when these drugs are used.

<u>Hyperstimulus and Hypertonus</u>

Hyperstimulus and hypertonus are associated with induction/augmentation, supine position, spontaneous labor, abruptio placentae, amnionitis, and use of illicit drugs. Hyperstimulus is usually defined as uterine contractions that occur more frequently than every 2 minutes; uterine relaxation < 30 seconds between contractions; and/or uterine contractions that continue longer than 90 seconds. Hypertonus usually is defined as elevated resting tone or peak pressure of the uterine contraction > 80 mm Hg or both. Abruptio placentae often is associated with hypertonus and hyperstimulus of either known or unknown etiology. The benefits of maternal hydration and tocolysis in the presence of excessive uterine activity warrant consideration. Terbutaline is used to treat hypertonus and hyperstimulation, especially when fetal compromise is present. This treatment is frequently termed intrauterine resuscitation (Simpson & Creehan, 1996).

Categories and Characteristics of Contractions

Although many terms are used to describe labor variations, the uterus basically contracts in one of three ways. <u>Normal</u> contractions are recognized more easily than <u>subnormal</u> and <u>abnormal</u> contractions, which are difficult to differentiate (Ueland, 1993). The tocodynamometer and IUPC, in combination with palpation and vaginal examination, may be used to assess uterine activity. The characteristics of these three types of uterine contractions are listed in Table 3-2.

Characteristics of Uterine Contractions

Normal Labor Characteristics

1. Fundal origin and dominance
2. Coordinated
3. 2-5 per 10-minute frequency
4. 45-90 second duration
5. 40-60 mm Hg first-stage intensity
6. 70-80 mm Hg late first-stage & second-stage intensity

7. Tonus
   a. 5-12 mm Hg without stimulation
   b. 20 mm Hg may be reached when Pitocin is used
8. Fundus at peak not indentible
9. Presenting part is tightly applied to cervix

Subnormal (Hypotonic) Labor

1. Fundal dominance
2. Less than 2-5 per 10-minute frequency
3. Less than 30 seconds duration
4. Less than 40 mm Hg intensity
5. Fundus at peak is indentible
6. Cervix at peak is not tightly applied to presenting part
7. Usually responds well to oxytocin augmentation

Abnormal Labor

1. No fundal dominance
2. Less frequent (usually)
3. Less intense (usually)
4. Mixed with subnormal and normal
5. Ineffective in dilatation and effacement
6. Fundus at peak may or may not be indentible
7. Cervix at peak is loosely applied to presenting part; room for examining finger

Table 3-2. Characteristics of uterine contractions associated with normal labor and variations in labor. (Klavin et al., 1977; May & Mahlmeister, 1994; Ueland, 1993)

Assessment of Uterine Activity

- Resting tone.
- Duration of contractions.
- Intensity of contractions.
- Frequency of contractions.
- Cervical changes as appropriate.
- Presence of factors affecting uterine contractions (e.g., maternal historical and physiologic data).
- Changes in uterine activity in response to interventions.

126

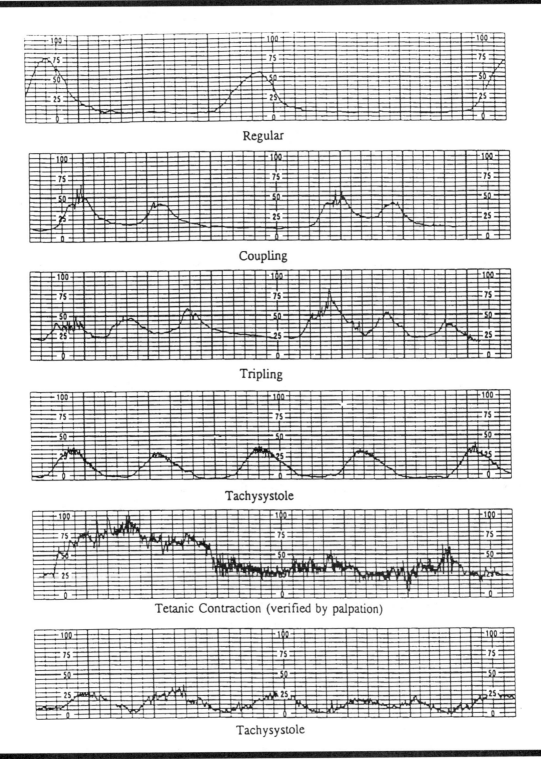

Regular

Coupling

Tripling

Tachysystole

Tetanic Contraction (verified by palpation)

Tachysystole

Figure 3-27. Samples of uterine activity representing a regular uterine contraction pattern and variations.

127

Monitoring the Preterm Pregnant Patient

"Interpreting FHR tracings from preterm fetuses requires knowledge of the underlying physiological changes related to fetal development" (Eganhouse & Burnside, 1992). A mature fetus as compared to a preterm fetus generally will possess characteristics including a decrease in baseline FHR to range between 110 and 150 bpm, an increase in LTV, an increase in the number and amplitude of accelerations, and pronounced changes in the appearance of the FHR tracing with fetal rest and state changes (Castillo et al., 1989; Naef et al., 1994; Pillai & James, 1990; Schifrin & Clement, 1990).

Physiology

The SNS dominates the FHR response until approximately 28 weeks of gestation when the PSNS overtakes the sympathetic control. Thus, an FHR baseline rate of 150-160 bpm is considered normal in a preterm fetus. The dominance of the FHR control by the PSNS slows the baseline FHR with increased gestational age. FHR accelerations can be seen as early as 24 weeks, yet these accelerations may usually only increase 10 bpm above the FHR baseline sustained for 10 seconds. These "preterm" accelerations, as they are often referred to (Ikuo, Akio, & Taro, 1992; Pillai & James, 1990), are seen more frequently than the "standard" acceleration of 15 bpm above the FHR baseline sustained for 15 seconds. In addition, decelerations lasting 10-20 seconds are common in low-risk fetuses between 20-30 weeks of gestation (Pillai & James, 1990). Fetal movement in these preterm fetuses may even elicit small decelerations instead of accelerations (Schifrin & Clement, 1990).

Baseline FHR

FHR reactivity of the fetus increases dramatically after 32 weeks of gestation. Current guidelines mandate that a fetus demonstrate reactivity by accelerating 15 bpm above the baseline for 15 seconds (Castillo et al., 1989; Eganhouse & Burnside, 1992; Murray, 1996). Exclusive use of these criteria increases the likelihood of false nonreactive nonstress tests for preterm fetuses, with some studies showing a rate of false test as high as 31.9% (Phelan et al., 1991). Yet, modifying the criteria for nonstress tests to accelerations of 10 bpm above baseline sustained for 10 seconds may be adequate for the preterm fetus to have a reactive strip. In addition to modifying the baseline parameters, the time element is extended to 60-90 minutes instead of the routine 20 minutes (Brown & Patrick, 1981; Castillo et al., 1989; Ikuo et al., 1992). In addition to the accelerations, reactivity of the preterm fetus can be assessed by looking at LTV. Routinely, LTV less than 6 bpm is classified as decreased or minimal (AWHONN, 1993), yet in the preterm fetus, LTV reaching that level may not occur until around 32 weeks of gestation. More acceptable LTV parameters for the preterm fetus are shown to be greater than or equal to 4.5 bpm (Ikuo et al., 1992; Natale, Nasello-Paterson, & Turliuk, 1985).

Uterine Activity

When assessing the preterm pregnancy, it is important to also look at uterine activity (UA). Because of the decreased sensitivity of tocodynamometers, detecting UA can be challenging for the perinatal professional. Therefore, it is most appropriate to incorporate the skill of uterine palpation to any professional's repertoire. Uterine activity may escalate in the 24 hours prior to the onset of preterm labor (Eganhouse & Burnside, 1992; Morrison, 1992; Newman, Campbell, & Stramm, 1990). This requires the nurse to understand key concepts regarding the assessment of preterm UA.

- Preterm contractions are often painless.
- Low amplitude high frequency (LAHF) contractions are an early sign of increasing UA (Eganhouse & Burnside, 1992).
- Perceived UA increases 24 hours before the onset of preterm labor (PTL).
- Standard tocodynamometers may not be sensitive enough to detect/record UA in preterm gestation (Eganhouse & Burnside, 1992; Naef et al., 1994).

Summary

Interpretation of the FHR is an important, yet challenging task, considering all the data that are available. Interpretation of the FHR characteristics includes: the baseline rate and its associated changes; variability; undulating patterns; rhythm and dysrhythmia recognition; and periodic and nonperiodic changes. In addition to the FHR, uterine activity also is an important parameter to assess and interpret. Many different factors, including hydration, maternal anxiety, maternal position, drugs, and medications can affect uterine activity. Length of gestation also plays a key role in the variances of interpretation of both the FHR and uterine activity. Interpretation requires a knowledge of maternal and fetal physiology to understand what the fetus and the maternal system are demonstrating, as well as knowledge regarding fetal monitoring techniques. Chapter 4 will continue with collaborative diagnosis and interventions based on these interpretation skills.

REFERENCES

Abitbol, M. (1985). Supine position in labor and associated fetal heart rate changes. Obstetrics and Gynecology, 65(4), 481-486.

Afriat, C. (1989). Electronic fetal monitoring. Rockville, MD: Aspen Publication.

Afriat, C. M. (1996). Intrapartum fetal monitoring. In K. R. Simpson & P. Creehan (Eds.), Perinatal Nursing (pp. 187-225). Philadelphia: Lippincott-Raven.

ACOG. (1995a). Dystocia and the augmentation of labor, ACOG Technical Bulletin No. 218. Washington, DC: Author.

ACOG. (1995b). Fetal heart rate patterns: Monitoring, interpretation, and management, ACOG Technical Bulletin No. 207. Washington, DC: Author.

ACOG. (1991). Induction and augmentation of labor, ACOG Technical Bulletin Number 157. Washington, DC: Author.

Arnold-Aldea, S.A., & Parer, J. (1990). Fetal cardiovascular physiology. In R.D. Eden & F.H. Bowhm (Eds.), Assessment and care of the fetus: Physiological, clinical and medicological principles. Norwalk, CT: Appleton & Lange.

AWHONN. (1993). Fetal heart monitoring principles and practices. Washington, DC: Author.

Baxi, L., & Petrie, R. (1987). Pharmacologic effects of labor: Effects of drugs on dystocia, labor, and uterine activity. Clinical Obstetrics and Gynecology, 30(1), 19-32.

Bowes, W. (1989). Clinical aspects of normal and abnormal labor. In R. K. Creasy & R. Resnik (Eds.), Maternal fetal medicine: Principles and practice (pp. 510-544). Philadelphia: W. B. Saunders Company.

Brown, R., & Patrick, J. (1981). The nonstress test: How long is enough? American Journal of Obstetrics and Gynecology, 141, 646-651.

Cabaniss, M. (1993). Fetal monitoring interpretation. Philadelphia, PA: Lippincott-Raven Publication.

Carlson, J., Diehl, J., Sachtleben-Murray, M., McRae, M., Fenwick, L., & Friedman, E. (1986). Maternal positioning during parturition in normal labor. Obstetrics and Gynecology, 68(4), 443-447.

Castillo, R., Devoe, L., Arthur, M., Searle, N., Metheny, W., & Ruedrich, D. (1989). The preterm nonstress test: Effects of gestational age and length of study. American Journal of Obstetrics and Gynecology, 160, 172-175.

Cohen, W. R., Acker, D. B., & Friedman, E. A. (Eds.) (1989). Management of labor (2nd ed.). Rockville, MD: Aspen.

Eden, R. (1989). Standards of care for the postdate pregnancy. Contemporary OB/GYN, 34(2), 39-55.

Eganhouse, D., & Burnside, S. (1992). Nursing assessment and responsibilities in monitoring the preterm pregnancy. Journal of Obstetric, Gynecologic, and Neonatal Nursing, 21(5), 355-363.

Elkington, K.W. (1991). At the water's edge: Where obstetrics and anesthesia meet, Clinical commentary. Obstetrics & Gynecology, 77(2), 304-308.

Fenwick, L., & Simpkin, P. (1987). Maternal positioning to prevent or relieve dystocia in labor. Clinical Obstetrics and Gynecology, 30, 83-89.

Freeman, R. K., Garite, T. J., & Nageotte, M. P. (1991). Fetal heart rate monitoring (2nd ed.). Baltimore: Williams & Wilkins.

Friedman, E. (1978). Labor: Clinical evaluation and management (2nd ed.). New York: Appleton-Century-Crofts.

Friedman, E. (1989). Failure to progress during labor. Contemporary OB/GYN, 34(6), 42-52.

Garfield, R. (1987). Cellular and molecular bases for dystocia. Clinical Obstetrics and Gynecology, 30, 3-18.

Grylack, L., Chu, S., & Scanlog, J. (1984). Use of intravenous fluids before cesarean section: Effects on perinatal glucose, insulin, and sodium homeostasis. Obstetrics & Gynecology, 63(5), 654-658.

Hammacher, K. (1969). The clinical significance of cardiotocography. In P. Huntingford, K. Huter, & E. Salez (Eds.), Perinatal medicine, 1st European Congress, Berlin (p. 81).

Hohn, A., & Stanton, R. (1992). The cardiovascular system. In A. Fanaroff & R. Martin (Eds.) Neonatal-perinatal medicine: Diseases of the fetus and infant (5th ed.). St. Louis, MO: Mosby-Year Book.

Hon, E. H. (1975). An introduction to fetal heart rate monitoring (2nd ed.). Los Angeles: USC School of Medicine.

Huszar, G., & Roberts, J. M. (1982). Biochemistry and pharmacology of the myometrium and labor: Regulation at the cellular and molecular levels. American Journal of Obstetrics and Gynecology, 142, 225.

Ikuo, S., Akio, I., & Taro, T. (1992). Longitudinal measurement of fetal heart rate (FHR) monitoring in second trimester. Early Human Development, 29, 251-257.

Klavin, M., Laver, A., & Boscola, M. (1977). Clinical concepts of fetal heart rate monitoring, Andover, MA: Hewlett-Packard Company.

Krebs, H. B., Petres, R. E., & Dunn, L. J. (1983). Intrapartum fetal heart rate monitoring VIII. Atypical variable deceleration. American Journal of Obstetrics and Gynecology, 145, 297-305.

Lederman, R.P., Lederman, E., Work, Jr., B.A., & McCann, D.S. (1978). The relationship of maternal anxiety, plasma catecholamines, and plasma cortisol to progress in labor. American Journal of Obstetrics and Gynecology, 135(5), 495-500.

Lederman, R.P., Lederman, E., Work, B., & McCann, D. S. (1985). Anxiety and epinephrine in multiparous women in labor: Relationship to duration of labor and fetal heart rate pattern. American Journal of Obstetrics and Gynecology, 153(8), 870-877.

Martin, C. (1982). Physiology and clinical use of fetal heart rate variability. Clinics in Perinatology, 9(2), 339.

Mattson, S., & Smith, J. (1993). AWHONN core curriculum for maternal-newborn nursing. Philadelphia: W.B. Saunders.

May, K., & Mahlmeister, L. (1994). Comprehensive maternity nursing. Philadelphia: Lippincott-Raven Publication.

Mondanlou, H., & Freeman, R. K. (1982). Sinusoidal fetal heart rate pattern: Its definition and clinical significance. American Journal of Obstetrics and Gynecology, 142, 1033.

Morrison, J. (1992). Assessment and management of preterm labor, Armed Forces District Conference (Statement). Norfolk, VA.

Morton, K.E., Jackson, M.C., & Gillmer, M.D.G. (1985). A comparison of the effects of four intravenous solutions for the treatment of ketonuria during labour. British Journal of Obstetrics and Gynaecology, 92, 473-479.

Murray, M. (1996). Antepartal and intrapartal fetal monitoring. Albuquerque, NM: Learning Resources International, Inc.

Myers, R. E. (1975). Maternal psychological stress and fetal asphyxia: A study in the monkey. American Journal of Obstetrics & Gynecology, 122(1), 47-59.

NAACOG. (1990). Fetal heart rate auscultation. OGN Nursing Practice Resource. Washington, DC: Author.

Naef, R., Morrison, J., Washburne, J., McLaughlin, B., Perry, K., & Roberts, W. (1994). Assessment of fetal well-being using the nonstress test in the home setting. Obstetrics & Gynecology, 84(3), 424-426.

Natale, R., Nasello-Paterson, C., & Turliuk, R. (1985). Longitudinal measurements of fetal breathing, body movements, heart rate, and heart rate accelerations and deceleration at 24 to 32 weeks of gestation. American Journal of Obstetrics and Gynecology, 151, 256.

Newman, R., Campbell, B., & Stramm, S. (1990). Objective tocodynamometry identifies labor onset earlier than subjective maternal perception. Obstetrics and Gynecology, 76, 1089-1092.

Parer, J. (1983). Handbook of fetal heart monitoring. Philadelphia: W. B. Saunders Company.

Parer, J. T. (1989). Fetal heart rate. In R. K. Creasy & R. Resnik (Eds.), Maternal fetal medicine: Principles and practice (p. 314). Philadelphia: W. B. Saunders Company.

Parer, J. T. (1997). Handbook of fetal heart rate monitoring (2nd Ed.). Philadelphia: W. B. Saunders Company.

Paul, R., Petrie, R., Rabello, Y., & Mueller, E. (1985). Fetal intensive care. Wallingford, CT: Corometrics Medical Systems.

Perkins, R. (1987). Fetal dystocia. Clinical Obstetrics and Gynecology, 30(1), 56-68.

Petrie, R. (Ed.). (1986). Intrapartum fetal monitoring. Clinical Obstetrics and Gynecology, 29.

Petrie, R. (1991). Intrapartum fetal evaluation. In S. Bagge, J. Neibyl, & J. Simpson (Eds.), Obstetrics: Normal and problem pregnancies (2nd ed.) (p. 457). New York: Churchill Livingstone.

Pillai, M., & James, D. (1990). The development of fetal heart rate patterns during normal pregnancy, Obstetrics & Gynecology, 76, 812-816.

Rosen, M., & Dickinson, J. (1993). The paradox of electronic fetal monitoring: More data may not enable us to predict or prevent infant neurologic morbidity. American Journal of Obstetrics and Gynecology, 168 (3.1), 745-751.

Schifrin, B. S., & Clement, D. (1990). Why fetal monitoring remains a good idea. Contemporary OB/GYN, 35, 70-86.

Schifrin, B. S., & Cohen, W.R. (1989). Labor's dysfunctional lexicon. Obstetrics and Gynecology, 74 (1), 121-124.

Simpkin, P. (1986). Stress, pain, and catecholamines in labor: Part 1. A review. Birth, 13(4), 227-232.

Simpson, K., & Creehan, P. (1996). Perinatal nursing. Philadelphia, PA: Lippincott-Raven Publication.

Singhi, S.C., & Chookang, E. (1984). Maternal fluid overload labour; transplacental hyponatremia and risk of transient neonatal tachypnea in term infants. Archives of Disease in Childhood, 59, 1155-1158.

133

Society of Obstetricians and Gynaecologists of Canada (SOGC). (1995). SOGC Policy Statement: Fetal health surveillance in labour. Journal of SOGC, 17(9), 865-901.

Tucker, S. (1992). Pocket guide to fetal monitoring (2nd ed.). St. Louis: Mosby Year Book.

Tucker, S. M. (1996). Fetal monitoring and assessment (3rd ed.). St. Louis: Mosby.

Ueland, K. (1993). Induction of labor and management of normal and abnormal labor. In J. J. Bonica & J. McDonald (Eds.), Principles and practice of obstetric analgesia and anesthesia (2nd ed.). Philadelphia: F.A. Davis

Welt, S. (1984). The fetal heart rate W-sign. Obstetrics and Gynecology, 63, 405.

BIBLIOGRAPHY

Adair, R. (1993). Fetal monitoring with adenosine administration. <u>Annals of Emergency Medicine,</u> <u>22</u>(12), 158.

Afriat, C. M. (1996). Intrapartum fetal monitoring. In K. R. Simpson & P. Creehan (Eds.), <u>Perinatal</u> <u>Nursing</u> (pp. 187-225). Philadelphia: Lippincott-Raven.

Arabin, B., Lorenz, U., Ruttgers, H., & Kubli, F. (1988). Course and predictive value of fetal heart rate parameters. <u>American Journal of Perinatology, 5</u>(3), 272-277.

Beall, M., & Paul, R. (1986). Artifacts, blocks, and arrhythmias: Confusing nonclassical heart rate tracings. <u>Clinical Obstetrics and Gynecology, 29,</u>(1) 83-94.

Blanch, G., Walkinshaw, S., & Walsh, K. (1994). Cardioversion of fetal tachyarrhythmia with adenosine. <u>Lancet, 344,</u> 1646.

Chan, F., Woo, S., Ghosh, A., Tang, M., & Lam, C. (1990). Prenatal diagnosis of congenital fetal arrhythmias by simultaneous pulsed doppler velocimetry of the fetal abdominal aorta and inferior vena cava. <u>Obstetrics and Gynecology, 76</u>(2), 200-205.

Chez, B. F., & Harvey, C. (1994). <u>Essentials of electronic fetal heart monitoring</u> (2nd ed.). Videotape series: Association of Women's Health, Obstetric and Neonatal Nurses (AWHONN). Baltimore, MD: Williams and Wilkins.

Danforth, D. N., & Ueland, K. (1986). Physiology of uterine action. In D. N. Danforth & J. R. Scott (Eds.), <u>Obstetrics and Gynecology</u> (5th ed.). Philadelphia: J.B. Lippincott.

Harvey, C., & Chez, B. F. (1996). <u>Critical concepts in fetal heart rate monitoring</u> (2nd ed.). Videotape series: Association of Women's Health, Obstetric and Neonatal Nurses (AWHONN). Baltimore, MD: Williams and Wilkins.

Hon, E. H. (1963). The classification of fetal heart rate. A revised working classification. <u>Obstetrics</u> <u>and Gynecology, 22,</u> 137.

Katz, M., Goodyear, K., & Creasy, R. K. (1990). Early signs and symptoms of preterm labor. <u>American</u> <u>Journal of Obstetrics and Gynecology, 162,</u> 1150-1153.

Kubo, T., Inaba, J., Shigemitsu, S., & Akatsuka, T. (1987). Fetal heart variability indices and the accuracy of variability measurements. <u>American Journal of Perinatology, 4</u>(3), 179-186.

Martin, C. (1978). Regulation of the fetal heart rate and genesis of FHR patterns. <u>Seminars in</u> <u>Perinatology, 2</u>(2), 131-146.

Murray, M. (1988). <u>Antepartal and intrapartal fetal monitoring</u>. Washington, DC: NAACOG.

Myers, R.E., & Myers, S.E. (1979). Use of sedative, analgesic, and anesthetic drugs during labor and delivery: Bane or boon? American Journal of Obstetrics and Gynecology, 133(1), 83-104.

NAACOG. (1989). Nursing responsibilities in implementing intrapartum fetal heart rate monitoring (Statement). Washington, DC: Author.

Petrie, R. (Ed.). (1986). Intrapartum fetal monitoring. Clinical Obstetrics and Gynecology, 29, 1.

Phelan, J. (1992). Legal aspects of C-section: Is the jury in?, Armed Forces District Conference (Statement). Norfolk, VA.

Quirk, J., & Miller, F. (1986). FHR tracing characteristics that jeopardize the diagnosis of fetal well-being. Clinical Obstetrics and Gynecology, 29(1), 12-22.

Ross, M., & Hayashi, R. (1984). How can we use oxytocin more effectively? Contemporary OB/GYN, 25, 139-146.

Schifrin, B. S. (1985). Exercises in fetal monitoring, Vol. 1. Los Angeles: BPM, Inc.

Schmidt, J. (1987). Documenting EFM events. Perinatal Press, 10, 79-81.

Schneider, E. P., & Tropper, P. J. (1986). The variable deceleration, prolonged deceleration, and sinusoidal fetal heart rate. Clinical Obstetrics and Gynecology, 29(1), 64-72.

Ueland, K., & Ueland, F. R. (1986). Dystocia due to abnormal uterine action. In D. N. Danforth & J. R. Scott (Eds.), Obstetrics and gynecology (5th ed.). Philadelphia: J.B. Lippincott.

Yeh, S., Forsythe, A., & Hon, E. (1973). Quantification of fetal heart beat-to-beat interval differences. Obstetrics and Gynecology, 41(3), 355-363.

CHAPTER 4: INTERVENTIONS

Introduction

The goal of fetal monitoring is to assess and promote maternal and fetal well-being. Both intrauterine and extrauterine influences can affect the fetal oxygenation status, in addition to an intact cardiovascular structure and neurologic system. By thoroughly assessing medical and obstetric history, risk factors, and physical assessment findings and systematically interpreting the fetal heart characteristics and uterine activity, the clinician has a better understanding of the fetal physiologic response to the perinatal period. Selection of appropriate interventions to maximize fetal oxygenation is based on these assessments and other relevant clinical information.

This chapter outlines principles of collaborative diagnosis and interventions following physiologic-based assessment and interpretation (Figure 4-1). The dynamic Physiologic Response Model (Figure 4-2) is used to conceptualize fetal status as a basis for interventions. The four goals of physiologic-based independent and collaborative interventions guide the discussions (Table 4-1). A brief discussion of acid-base assessment also is included. This chapter concludes with selected examples of interventions and an algorithm for fetal heart monitoring decisions (Figure 4-4).

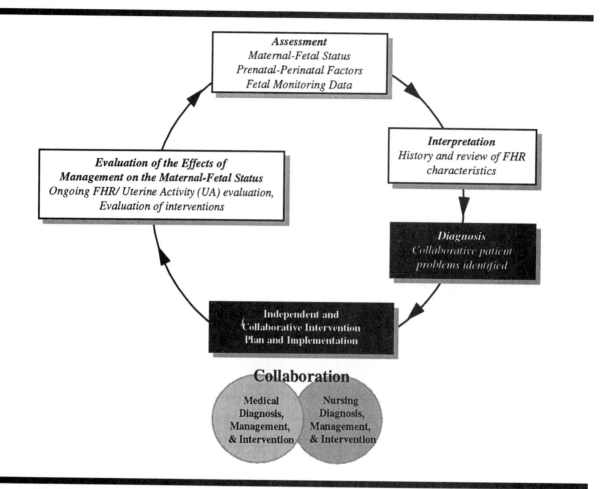

Figure 4-1. The nursing process and fetal heart monitoring: Interventions.

Systematic Interpretation of the FHR Pattern

Systematic interpretation of the fetal heart pattern includes reviewing both the uterine activity and fetal heart characteristics. The method of monitoring used will determine which characteristics can be assessed adequately. Systematic fetal monitoring assessment includes the following:

I. UTERINE ACTIVITY

- Frequency
- Duration
- Intensity
- Resting tone

II. BASELINE FHR CHARACTERISTICS

- Baseline rate
- Rhythm
- Variability
    - Long-term variability (LTV)
    - Short-term variability (STV)
- Undulations

III. BASELINE CHANGES

- Periodic patterns
    - Accelerations
    - Decelerations
        - Early
        - Variables
        - Late
        - Combined Decelerations
- Nonperiodic patterns
    - Accelerations
    - Decelerations
    - Variables
    - Prolonged

(Hon, 1975; Martin, 1982; Murray, 1988; NAACOG, 1991; Parer, 1989; Petrie, 1991; ACOG, 1995a)

A systematic approach to the interpretation of fetal monitoring data in light of the entire patient picture encourages a more complete evaluation. While the experienced clinician may perform many parts of the assessment simultaneously, based on prior knowledge and experience, each practitioner is encouraged to address all of the fetal heart characteristics and uterine activity when planning interventions.

A brief review or discussion of the terms *reassuring patterns* and *nonreassuring patterns* may be helpful here. The terms reassuring and nonreassuring have been used to describe fetal monitoring patterns. In some cases, the terms have been used to describe particular characteristics of a pattern. However, in general, the terms are used more commonly to describe the fetal status or outcome. A reassuring pattern may be viewed as representing a fetus that demonstrates a favorable physiologic response during the perinatal period. Reassuring implies that the fetus may be assumed to have normal oxygen and acid base status (ACOG, 1995a). At the other end of the spectrum, a nonreassuring pattern may be viewed as a fetus demonstrating an implied nonreassuring or unfavorable physiologic response. Nonreassuring patterns, however, are "non-specific and cannot reliably predict whether a fetus will be well oxygenated, depressed or acidotic" (ACOG, 1995a, p. 4). In addition to hypoxemia, other factors may lead to a nonreassuring pattern. A nonreassuring fetal heart pattern implies that the clinician is not reassured by the findings, although the term allows for the occurrence of a positive outcome given the lack of ability to predict outcomes precisely (ACOG, 1994).

With appropriate interventions, the goal is to maximize the likelihood of favorable responses while addressing nonreassuring responses. When nonreassuring patterns occur, there is a need to further assess and to intervene. The Dynamic Physiologic Response Model provides a way of viewing patterns based on their characteristics. While the fetal heart rate patterns may change and may become more reassuring after interventions, this model is not intended to imply a continuum that fetuses will go through in a particular order. What is notable in this model is that normal features exist in the reassuring pattern; rate rhythm, variability, absence of decelerations and presence of accelerations. Early decelerations with normal features also are not associated with hypoxemia. As the pattern becomes nonreassuring, the variability is notably decreased or absent and often with additional changes from the normal baseline (e.g., tachycardia, bradycardia, decelerations). In addition, some fetal heart patterns may not be categorized as either reassuring or nonreassuring such as some dysrhythmias. Therefore, as previously emphasized, interventions are centered on addressing the specific physiologic responses whether the pattern is viewed as a reassuring/favorable or has a nonreassuring/unfavorable response.

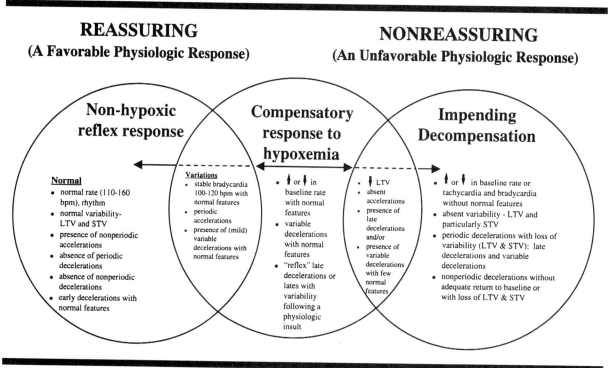

Figure 4-2. Alterations of FHR patterns by dynamic physiologic response.

Examples of nursing diagnoses that specifically address underlying physiology might include

- Alteration in fetal gas exchange related to umbilical cord compression, as evidenced by variable decelerations.

- Alteration in placental gas perfusion related to post-term gestation or placental degeneration, as evidenced by late decelerations and absent variability.

An example of a collaborative problem would be the "potential for fetal compromise."

Physiologic-Based Interventions

Interventions focus primarily on promoting adequate placental perfusion and oxygenation of the fetus, while also attempting to remove or minimize factors interfering with adequate fetal circulation with oxygenated blood. The four general physiologic goals of interventions are intended to

- Improve uterine blood flow
- Improve umbilical circulation
- Improve oxygenation
- Reduce uterine activity

Specific actions for each of these goals may reappear under more than one goal (Table 4-1). Maternal position change may have an impact on all four goals and is usually one of the first actions indicated. The choice of interventions will be based on the assessments, interpretations, and underlying pathophysiologic factors. Rather than implementing all actions universally, actions should be based on specific pathophysiology. If an unfavorable or nonreassuring pattern develops, already exists, or worsens, the interventions will increase in number and intensity to foster "intrauterine resuscitation."

Interventions to promote intrauterine resuscitation are important. Intrauterine resuscitation has been defined in various ways. Intrauterine resuscitation definitions and methods have ranged from infusion of sodium bicarbonate to the mother in the 1960s to the infusion of high glucose (>40%) solutions, ascorbic acid infusions and administration of oxygen in the 1970s; and finally, to actions that enhance uterine and umbilical blood flow for optimum oxygenation of the mother, and ultimately for the fetus, in the 1980s and 1990s (AWHONN, 1993; Jauniaux et al., 1994; Murray, 1996; Newman, Mitchell, & Wood, 1967). In this book, it is used to refer to a collection of patient-specific interventions that are used to address nonreassuring FHR characteristics or patterns to promote fetal oxygenation, and hopefully, the return of reassuring FHR characteristics or patterns. Nonreassuring FHR characteristics and patterns can be related to maternal or fetal insults or both. If a nonreassuring FHR pattern does not return to a reassuring pattern despite appropriate interventions, additional measures to correct the causative factor(s) and resuscitate the fetus. Operative interventions with a compromised fetus may not always be the most appropriate intervention. If intrauterine resuscitation is used, resulting in the recovery to a reassuring FHR pattern, labor can continue without the added stress of emergency operative delivery for both fetus and mother. Yet, if despite all the interventions, including measures to resuscitate the fetus in utero, are unsuccessful, operative delivery may be necessary.

Interventions to maximize fetal perfusion and oxygenation should continue until appropriate changes in fetal status (as evidenced by FHR characteristics and/or fetal blood gas values) have been achieved or birth takes place (Table 4-1).

Goals of Physiologic Interventions

Improve Uterine Blood Flow
- Maternal position change
- Hydration
- Anxiety reduction
- Medication

Improve Oxygenation
- Maternal position change
- Maternal oxygen
- Maternal breathing techniques

Improve Umbilical Circulation
- Maternal position change
- Vaginal manipulation
- Amnioinfusion

Reduce Uterine Activity
- Maternal position change
- Hydration
- Modified pushing
- Medication (e.g., discontinue or decrease rate of labor-stimulating drug infusion)

Table 4-1. Four goals and interventions associated with maximizing fetal perfusion and oxygenation. These interventions may include both independent nursing action and collaborative actions. (Refer to Figure 4-1)

Additional Measures

In addition to interventions to promote fetal perfusion and oxygenation, other actions focus on instrumentation and further assessment of fetal response to labor, interventions, or both. These measures may be used to further clarify the fetal status or response to interventions. Ongoing assessments and patient responses should be clearly documented and communicated to other health-care providers.

Monitoring actions may include

- Verification of monitoring data.
- Troubleshooting the monitoring method in use.
- Changing to a new method of monitoring.

Additional collaborative assessment includes:

- Fetal/newborn acid-base assessment
    - Fetal stimulation (e.g., scalp acoustic)
    - Fetal capillary blood sampling (assist MD)
    - Cord blood sampling

- Real-time ultrasound.
- Kleihauer-Betke test or APT test.
- Maternal vital signs.
- Vaginal examination for labor progress, presenting part assessment, and umbilical cord.

Fetal/Newborn Acid-Base Assessment

Although this course focuses on fetal heart monitoring, it is important to understand fetal acid-base monitoring as it is often used as an adjunct to fetal monitoring. To understand and interpret acid-base values, it is necessary to understand normal glucose metabolism. A brief overview of normal glucose metabolism, physiologic and pathophysiologic factors affecting acid-base status, as well as indirect and direct methods of assessing this status follows.

Normal Glucose Metabolism

In normal cellular glucose metabolism, energy is released during glycolysis (splitting) of the glucose molecules and during the oxidation of the end-products of glycolysis. During an early anaerobic phase of carbohydrate metabolism, glucose is initially converted to pyruvic acid through a series of chemical reactions. Eventually, through the Krebs cycle, chemical reactions within the cell mitochondria result in carbon dioxide and hydrogen atom formation. Subsequently, oxidation of the hydrogen atoms occurs. Adenosine triphosphate (ATP), which is energy for use by the cells, is formed during these processes with the largest amount formed during oxidation of the hydrogen atoms (Guyton, 1992).

During anaerobic metabolism, when oxygen is not available for the oxidation of the hydrogen atoms, cellular oxidation of the hydrogen cannot take place. Small amounts of energy may be released through the initial glucose breaking down into pyruvic acid. With extended periods of decrease in oxygen, the end-products of chemical reactions build up. The build-up of hydrogen and pyruvic acid leads to lactic acid formation through chemical reactions. In the absence of oxygen, lactic acid cannot be broken down and it accumulates resulting in metabolic acidemia. With the addition of oxygen (at the cellular level), lactic acid is then converted resulting in formation of carbon dioxide which enters the umbilical arteries and is transported into the maternal circulation for excretion through the maternal system. The process of reversing metabolic acidosis with adequate oxygenation can take as long as 20-30 minutes or longer, depending on the degree of acidosis. Therefore, fetuses with metabolic acidosis in utero may exhibit decreased variability, possible loss of variability, neurologic compromise, and even intrauterine fetal death.

When umbilical cord compression or occlusion occurs, CO_2 produced by lactic acid conversion, cannot be removed from the fetal circulation and results in a buildup of CO_2. The excess CO_2 is hydrolyzed and carbonic acid is formed resulting in respiratory acidosis. However, respiratory acidosis is easily reversed in utero when the umbilical cord compression is released, as the CO_2 is quickly diffused into the maternal circulation for excretion through the maternal system.

Physiologic and Pathophysiologic Factors Affecting Intrapartum Acid-Base Assessment

- Fetal acid-base status depends on maternal regulation and transplacental transfer of gases.

- Fetal pH is slightly lower than the maternal pH.

- Mild maternal metabolic acidemia may develop during labor due to muscular activity, catecholamine release, or relative starvation.

- During prolonged second stage the fetus may develop respiratory acidemia.

- Accumulated carbonic acids are excreted rapidly across the placenta if blood flow is restored in a reasonable period of time.

- Repeated umbilical cord compression may cause fetal respiratory acidemia. With adequate cord release, a healthy fetus will be able to resuscitate itself in utero. Depending on the duration of the temporary insult, the fetus will excrete carbon dioxide across the placenta if allowed sufficient time.

- Metabolic acidemia in the fetus results from an accumulation of noncarbonic acid formed by anaerobic glycolysis (lactic acid). This is secondary to inadequate levels of oxygen (hypoxemia).

- Accumulated noncarbonic acid is excreted across the placenta mostly by fetal kidneys at a far slower rate, requiring hours rather than seconds, even if sufficient oxygenation is restored. Therefore, sustained hypoxemia may be associated with the development of metabolic acidosis.

- A mixture of respiratory and metabolic acidosis may occur.

Direct and indirect methods may be used to provide additional information about the acid-base status of the fetus and newborn. These will be reviewed briefly in this section. Further references are provided and recommended; hospital guidelines and protocols should be referred to and followed when implementing these procedures.

Indirect Methods of Acid-Base Assessment

The indirect methods used to evaluate the fetal status will attempt to elicit a reactive response which is predictive of a normoxic fetus (generally a pH ≥ 7.20) with a normoxic central nervous system. The stimulus used to elicit the reactive response (acceleration of 15 bpm amplitude with a duration of 15 seconds) may be acoustic stimulation, abdominal palpation stimulation (Freeman, Garite, & Nageotte, 1991), or scalp stimulation via vaginal examination (Figure 4-3). While reactivity is associated with normoxia or fetal well-being, the absence of an acceleration does not diagnose acidemia or predict fetal compromise. Further observation and assessment measures are indicated. Selection of assessment measures is based on the maternal-fetal history, labor progress, and maternal status.

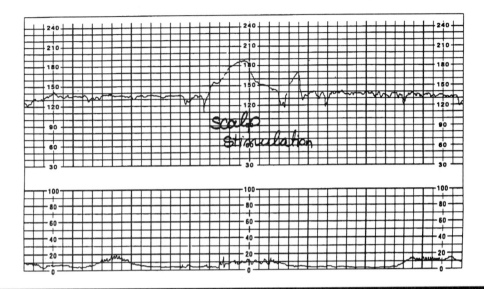

Figure 4-3. Scalp stimulation with vaginal examination elicits an acceleration to 190 from baseline of 135 to 140 bpm.

Decision algorithms vary and may resemble the following (Table 4-2):

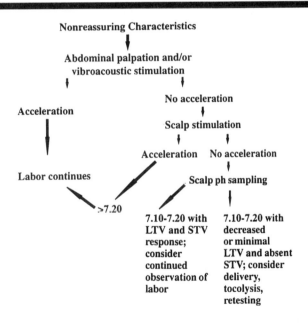

Table 4-2. Example of Decision Algorithm for Assessing Fetal Acid-Base Status. (Adapted from Gilstrap, Leveno, Burris, Williams, & Little, 1989; Sykes, Johnson, & Ashworth, 1982)

Direct Methods

When the fetal status is unclear via auscultation or the EFM tracing, or when confusing fetal heart and uterine activity patterns exist, blood sampling may provide additional information. Fetal capillary sampling is obtained via vaginal access for a scalp blood sample. Umbilical blood sampling can be obtained via in utero methods (cordocentesis or percutaneous umbilical blood sampling-PUBS) but is more commonly obtained at delivery to provide retrospective information as well as newborn stabilization information (Sonek & Nicolaides, 1994).

More definitive and objective markers for fetal asphyxia are currently being evaluated. For example, one study found that nucleated red blood cells (NRBC) may assist in the timing of fetal asphyxia (Phelan, Ahn, Martin, 1995). NRBC are not normally found in the neonate, yet, when asphyxia occurred, distinctive NRBC patterns could be identified that corresponded to the observed intrapartum FHR pattern. These researchers concluded that cord blood NRBC may assist in the timing of neurologic injury of the neonate.

Fetal Scalp Sampling

When the auscultated FHR characteristics or EFM pattern interpretation is inconclusive, and the fetus has not responded to stimuli, further assessment may be indicated. Although there may be some variation of preference by institution and practitioner, the following indications often are used by those who employ fetal scalp sampling. In cases of persistent nonreassuring patterns implying fetal or maternal compromise, when acidemia cannot be ruled out, maternal intervention or expedient delivery may be indicated (ACOG, 1995a). The steps of fetal scalp sampling are provided in manuals and texts, as well as by manufacturers who produce kits for sampling. Although the steps are simple, the actual sampling techniques involve rupture of the membranes and require appropriate care and experience. See Appendix 4a for a discussion of fetal scalp sampling technique.

Indications for Fetal Scalp Sampling

- Unexplained decreased or minimal LTV/absent STV without periodic or nonperiodic changes.
- Undulating or sinusoidal pattern of unknown origin.
- Late decelerations with absent or decreasing STV and LTV.
- Abnormal or unusual fetal heart patterns/characteristics.

Contraindications for Fetal Scalp Sampling

The principal relative contraindications for this procedure are listed below. Limiting factors may include availability of equipment and practitioners experienced in fetal scalp sampling. While the risks and benefits of this procedure are controversial, the relative contraindications also must be considered.

Relative Contraindications for Fetal Scalp Sampling

- Fetal coagulopathy-actual or suspected (e.g., hemophilia, thrombocytopenia).
- Active maternal genital infections (e.g., herpes, group B streptococcus).
- Suspected or documented HIV.
- Chorioamnionitis.

Factors Affecting Sampling and Interpretation of Results

There are factors to be considered during the sampling process that may or may not be controlled by the skill of the practitioner obtaining the sample. Some factors to be considered in the sampling and interpretation of results include

- Presentation, position, station, dilation, effacement.
- Thick fetal hair.
- Equipment and resources available.
- Time lapse for filling the capillary tube.
- Machine calibration.
- Maternal acid-base balance-especially the complicated obstetric patient who may need to be simultaneously sampled for comparative evaluation with the fetus.
- Uterine activity at the time of sampling.
- Fetal trauma related to procedure (e.g., hemorrhage, abscess).
- Presence of meconium.
- Sampling in area of cephalhematoma and fontanels.
- Contamination of the sample.
- Cooperation of the mother.

Outcome and Interpretation

There are several different mean values and norms of scalp pH and blood gas values reported by investigators as well as reports of correlations with Apgar scores. This creates more discussion for broadening the scalp or umbilical cord pH value of 7.20 as the delineation between nonacidemia and acidemia (ACOG, 1995; Gilstrap et al., 1989).

- Fetal scalp pH between 7.15 and 7.25 in the second stage of labor may be unreliable in predicting the condition of the newborn at birth because of transitory respiratory acidosis.
- A fetal scalp pH greater than 7.15 is associated with a 1-minute Apgar score of more than 6 in 86% of newborns.
- A fetal scalp pH greater than 7.20 is associated with a 1-minute Apgar score of more than 6 in 94% of newborns.

147

When values below 7.20 or even 7.20-7.25 are obtained, interpretation factors to be considered include the following:

- Accuracy of sampling and measurement (e.g., presence of hair, caput, air contamination from slow blood flow, difficulty in equipment calibration or function, presence of meconium.

- Type of acidosis (e.g., respiratory, metabolic, or mixed).

- Relationship of the time of the sample to uterine contractions.

- Relationship of the time of the sample to FHR characteristics, patterns, stage of labor, and clinical circumstance.

Important Considerations in Fetal Scalp Sampling

Regardless of the pH value used as the delineation between nonacidemia and acidemia, it is more important to view the value in terms of a trend. The clinician must evaluate whether the pH is rising or falling. This perspective may be the most useful in evaluating both the tracing and the results of the scalp sampling in the clinical setting (International Federation of Gynecology and Obstetrics [IFGO], 1995). Furthermore, pH is a less satisfactory measure of acidemia than a combination of pH and base deficit because of variations of acidemia which may be present at the time of blood sampling (SOGC, 1995).

Umbilical Cord Blood Sampling

Analysis of umbilical cord blood gases has been useful in assessment of the fetal respiratory status and to quantify the extent of fetal acidemia. Blood gases provide a more objective means of excluding birth asphyxia, than the more subjective Apgar score. For the preterm infant, whose neurologic immaturity influences the Apgar score, the umbilical cord blood gases provide an unprejudiced assessment of the neonatal status (Dickinson, Erikson, Meyer, & Parisi, 1992). See Appendix 4b for a discussion of cord blood sampling technique. Normal ranges for umbilical cord blood values have been suggested in the literature (Table 4-3) (ACOG, 1995b; Yeoman, Hauth, Gilstrap, & Strickland, 1985).

Indications for Umbilical Cord Blood Sampling

- Nonreassuring fetal heart characteristics/tracing.
- Thick meconium.
- Low Apgar scores.
- Preterm birth.
- Forceps and vacuum extraction.
- Emergent cesarean deliveries (ACOG, 1995b).

Contraindications

- None.

148

Factors Affecting Sampling and Interpretation of Results

- Differences in methodology used, such as duration of procedure, air bubbles, etc.
- Differences in heparin concentration use such
    - biarbonate and pCO_2 show an inverse relationship with the volume of heparin used (Duerbeck, Chaffin, & Seeds, 1992).
- Sampling of venous versus arterial blood.

Normal Ranges for Umbilical Cord Blood

Cord Blood	pH	pCO_2(mm Hg)	pO_2 (mm Hg)	Bicarbonate (meq/L)
ARTERIAL	7.28	49.2	18.0	22.3
range	7.15-7.43	31.1-74.3	3.8-33.8	13.3-27.5
VENOUS	7.35	38.2	29.2	20.4
range	7.24-7.49	23.3-49.2	15.2-48.2	15.9-24.7

Table 4-3. Normal Ranges for Umbilical Cord Blood (ACOG, 1995b; Yeomans, Hauth, Gilstrap, & Strickland, 1985)

Significance of Deviation from Normal Values

Type of Acidosis	pH	pCO_2	HCO_3	Base Deficit
Respiratory	↓	↑	normal	normal
Metabolic	↓	normal	↓	↑
Mixed	↓	↑	↓	↑

Table 4-4. Significance of Deviation from Normal Values (ACOG, 1995b)

If a low 1-minute Apgar score accompanies a low pH value, the pCO_2, pO_2 and base deficit will assist in determining whether the insult is acute or chronic and respiratory, metabolic, or mixed acidemia (Table 4-4) (Fields, Entman, & Boehm, 1983). Finally, the terms fetal asphyxia or birth asphyxia frequently are used inappropriately or incorrectly. These terms should not be used in documentation and only refer to the clinical context of damaging acidemia, hypoxemia, and metabolic acidosis (ACOG, 1994).

Birth asphyxia has been associated with the following neonatal clinical signs (ACOG, 1994):

- Apgar score of 0 to 3 at $\geq$5 minutes.

- Central nervous system injury with alteration in consciousness and seizures.

- Signs of multisystem organ failure.

- pH < 7.00 on arterial cord blood sample.

- Base deficit greater than or equal to 16 (Gilstrap et al., 1989).

Interpretation of Acid-Base Values

There is much in the literature regarding interpretation of normal and metabolic, respiratory, or mixed acidemia blood values (ACOG, 1995b; Cabaniss, 1993; AWHONN, 1992; Simpson & Creehan, 1996; Winkler, Tucker, Owen, & Brumfeld, 1991). Values above 7.25 for scalp pH are considered to be normal, while values between 7.20 and 7.25 are considered borderline. Values below 7.20 for scalp pH are considered to be acidemia. For umbilical cord blood, normal mean arterial blood values ranging from 7.27 to 7.28 have been reported for term infants (ACOG, 1995b). Values for preterm infants are similar for pH with a range of 7.26 to 7.29 (ACOG, 1995b). Historically, cord blood pH values below 7.20 have been defined as acidemia. Values between 7.10 and 7.19 have been reported as lower ranges of normal values (Sykes, Molloy, Johnson, Ashworth, & Stirrat, 1982; Gilstrap et al., 1989). Blood pH values below 7.00 have been associated with adverse neonatal outcomes (including death) and more clearly represent a threshhold for significant or pathologic fetal acidemia (ACOG, 1995b; Gilstrap et al., 1989).

Although normal blood values are often described in ranges, it may be helpful to identify a number to be used as a frame of reference when evaluating cord blood values. In addition to pH, the pO_2, pCO_2, bicarbonate, and base deficit or excess values are often considered.

	Normal Values	Metabolic Acidemia	Respiratory Acidemia
pH	>7.10	<7.10	<7.10
pO_2 (mm Hg)	>20	<20	variable
pCO_2 (mm Hg)	<60	<60	>60
Bicarbonate (mEq./L)	>22	<22	<22
BD/BE (mEq./L)	<10/-10	>10/-10	<10/-10

As indicated by the values, a decreased pH reflects higher acid level and, therefore, acidemia. Plasma bicarbonate is one buffer that is used to raise pH levels. In metabolic acidosis, an excess of hydrogen ions are released. As a result, bicarbonate, a base is depleted (Cohen & Schifrin, 1983; Gimovsky, & Caritis, 1982). The decrease in base is reflected as an increased base deficit or decreased base excess. The base deficit or excess is not measured directly, but is calculated from the pH, pCO_2, and bicarbonate blood values.

150

Base deficit measures the amount of base buffer below normal levels. A large positive base deficit indicates that base buffers have been used to buffer acids, that sufficient base reserves are not present, and that metabolic acidosis is present. Base excess measures the amount of base buffers above normal levels. Therefore, a large negative base excess also indicates that base buffers have been used to buffer acids, that sufficient base reserves are not present, and that metabolic acidosis is present. The use of base deficit vs. base excess is often laboratory dependent; some laboratories measure base deficit and some measure base excess.

Regardless of what specific values are used, it is important to assess the trends of serial pH values obtained from scalp and cord blood values when assessing the situation for recovery.

Selected Interventions

A brief overview of interventions for selected fetal heart changes will be presented in this section. When dealing with *patterns or combinations of patterns* in the clinical setting, focusing on whether the pattern represents a "blood flow problem," an "oxygenation" problem, or both may be helpful when selecting interventions. All interventions listed under each category are not intended to be used each time a pattern appears. One primary intervention may be all that is required. For example, for a variable deceleration pattern, maternal position change may be all that is necessary. However, if other features exist with that pattern, such as absent STV, or if the initial intervention does not resolve the problem, further physiologic interventions may be required. Therefore, these lists are intended to suggest possible interventions and do not imply that all are required for each pattern or that no other steps are required. The selection of interventions is individualized based on observed maternal-fetal physiologic response.

Interventions for Baseline Rate

<u>Interventions for Tachycardia</u>

- Change maternal position.
- Hydrate.
- Medicate.
- Decrease or discontinue oxytocin, depending upon variability and other fetal heart characteristics.
- Decrease maternal temperature, if elevated.
- Assess possible drug use.
- Reduce anxiety; assist with breathing techniques.
- Administer oxygen mask per protocol.

When selecting interventions for tachycardia, the entire maternal-fetal "picture" is reviewed. Fetal heart and uterine activity characteristics are assessed, with underlying physiologic factors associated with the development of the tachycardia. Each of the following situations illustrates such an assessment.

When tachycardia appears with normal variability, without periodic or nonperiodic decelerations, and normal gestational age is present, the cause may be maternal fever. If the temperature is elevated, appropriate nursing, medical, and collaborative management of the cause of the fever is appropriate. Interventions should focus on eliminating the problem causing the fever. Position change may foster the umbilical blood flow while hydration, as indicated, might prevent or alleviate the effects of dehydration. Antipyretics also may be used.

When the fetus is exhibiting tachycardia in response to epinephrine stimulation, anxiety reduction measures may be helpful. Tachycardia resulting from maternal medications, such as Beta-sympathomimetics, may be expected and may not be entirely eliminated. Observation of maternal and fetal responses to the medications is warranted (e.g., pulse, FHR).

When tachycardia is a response to fetal hypoxia, further interventions and assessments are indicated. Tachycardia is a compensatory response to hypoxia. The focus of interventions will be on improving uterine blood flow, umbilical blood flow and oxygenation, and on decreasing uterine activity. When associated with variable or late decelerations and decreased variability, tachycardia may indicate chronic hypoxia requiring collaborative care and further interventions.

When tachycardia is the result of a cardiac abnormality or arrhythmia, medical management and collaborative care focus on the cause and effects of the tachycardia. Maternal positioning, oxygen administration, and other actions may be warranted, depending on the type and extent of the tachycardia. Fetal cardiac output is dependent on FHR and may be significantly decreased at rates over 200 bpm.

Interventions for Bradycardia

- Change maternal position.

- Hydrate.

- Perform vaginal manipulation to elevate presenting part.

- Administer maternal oxygen.

- Discontinue oxytocin.

- Modify pushing.

- Decrease uterine activity.

- Differentiate FHR from maternal heart rate.

As with tachycardia, the fetal and maternal assessments attempt to identify the physiologic reason for bradycardia. Technological artifact and maternal pulse should be ruled out. Further assessment to verify fetal well-being may include review of the gestational age, vaginal examination, fetal stimulation, or application of spiral electrode to assess STV.

When a stable bradycardic rate of 90-120 bpm, with average LTV and accelerations is seen, routine assessments and interventions may be the only actions warranted. Fetal maturation may be associated with a stable bradycardic rate such as this.

If maternal position is a factor in the development of a reflex bradycardia, position change is warranted to correct hypotension and increase uterine blood flow and/or increase umbilical cord flow. If hypoxic changes are evident, other actions to enhance uterine blood flow, improve umbilical circulation, improve oxygenation, and reduce uterine activity are necessary, particularly when other baseline changes, such as decreased or absent variability, occur.

Cardiac arrhythmias or dysrhythmias may be the underlying cause of bradycardia. In the presence of a cardiac conduction defect, hypoxia is not usually the cause of the bradycardia, especially in the absence of other nonreassuring FHR findings. Further evaluation and interventions as described in the previous section are warranted.

Interventions for Variability

Long-Term Variability (LTV)

    Interventions for Average LTV

When LTV is average, the intervention may be only to continue routine assessments and interventions, as the presence of LTV is a reassuring finding. Interventions will focus on maintaining the presence of variability and removing any additional stressors, such as cord compression, if present.

Interventions for Decreased LTV

- Change position.
- Hydrate.
- Discontinue oxytocin.
- Provide information and reduce anxiety.
- Change maternal breathing patterns.
- Assess medication influence, use of illicit drugs or alcohol.

When periods of decreased variability ($\downarrow$ LTV) occur prior to or following episodes of normal variability, the cause of the $\downarrow$ LTV may be fetal sleep or a medication effect. Continued assessments and routine care may be all that is warranted.

If the LTV is decreasing with other FHR changes, such as variable or late decelerations, or is decreasing while other FHR changes are occurring and normal causes have been ruled out, a blood flow problem (placental or cord), an oxygenation problem, or both may exist. Interventions will focus on increasing uterine blood flow and umbilical flow, improving oxygenation, and reducing uterine activity as indicated by the given pattern. Variability is a significant indicator of how well the fetus is tolerating a given stressor. Further actions, such as validating the monitoring data, changing to a spiral electrode for improved assessment of LTV and STV, and assessing fetal stimulation and/or fetal scalp pH, may be indicated to further evaluate fetal status.

If maternal hyperventilation occurs, the breathing pattern may be altered through effective coaching to slow breathing as well as administration of oxygen per mask at 8 L/minute.

Interventions for Marked/Saltatory LTV

- Change position.
- Hydrate.
- Discontinue oxytocin.
- Administer oxygen.
- Alter breathing/pushing.
- Provide information and reduce anxiety.
- Administer tocolytics.

Short-Term Variability (STV)

Interventions for Present STV

When present, STV provides reassurance about the oxygen reserves available and the functioning of the medulla oblongata and autonomic nervous system, particularly, the parasympathetic nervous system. When STV is present with other patterns, such as late or variable decelerations, it may indicate that oxygen reserves are still present, but interventions are warranted to remove or minimize the stressors.

Interventions for Absent STV

- Promote uterine or umbilical blood flow.
- Improve oxygenation.
- Reduce uterine activity.
- Rule out instrumentation error (artifact).
- Rule out drug/medication effect.
- Assess fetal status as indicated.
  -- scalp stimulation
  -- acoustic stimulation
  -- fetal scalp sampling
- Plan for delivery and management of neonate.

Undulating Patterns

Interventions for Undulating Patterns

When undulating patterns are observed, the etiology may range from a minor and temporary change due to analgesia or magnesium sulfate, to a more serious and persistent change due to anemia and severe hypoxia as in isoimmunization. These responses each warrant different interventions, although identification of a sinusoidal pattern versus a pseudosinusoidal pattern may be difficult. The interventions begin with a re-examination of the patient's history, as well as a physical assessment. The presence of STV is reassuring. Undulating patterns that do not exist prior to analgesic administration frequently can be attributed to the analgesic.

A true sinusoidal pattern associated with isoimmunization or placental abruption is nonreassuring. A history of Rh status and possible isoimmunization should be elicited. Signs and symptoms of abruption also should be assessed to include pain, vaginal bleeding, and an increase in uterine resting tone. Risk factors for abruption, such an abdominal trauma, rapid decompression of the uterus, and cocaine use, also should be evaluated.

155

Supportive measures for a true sinusoidal pattern include improving uterine blood flow and oxygenation. Additional interventions range from an expedient delivery to intrauterine fetal blood transfusion via cordocentesis.

Fetal Dysrhythmias

Interventions for Fetal Dysrhythmias

The types of fetal heart irregularities that can be identified are outlined in the rhythm section of Chapter 3. When an irregularity is detected, further assessment to determine etiology and severity is undertaken. An intermittent irregularity, with normal heart rate, average STV, and fetal reactivity often requires only observation and maintenance of uterine blood flow and oxygenation.

A persistent tachycardia with fixed R-wave to R-wave intervals or an absence of STV may require further ultrasound diagnosis and pharmacologic therapy, such as Digoxin. Notice that this problem is referred to as supraventricular tachycardia or SVT, a term not to be confused with short-term variability (STV).

In addition, the current maternal history may indicate chronic disease, such as systemic lupus erythematosus (SLE), drug use, or uncontrolled diabetes, as these may be associated with dysrhythmias. The etiology of and type of dysrhythmia will determine the intervention.

Variable Decelerations

Interventions for Variable Decelerations

- Change maternal position.
- Perform vaginal exam for prolapse cord or imminent delivery.
- Perform amnioinfusion.
- Provide information and reduce anxiety.
- Administer oxygen if associated with decreased variability.

The primary intervention to improve umbilical cord perfusion is maternal position change. Such changes are thought to decrease pressure on the umbilical cord and improve fetal and maternal blood flow. Maternal position changes are intended to either resolve or improve the variable deceleration pattern. It should be noted, however, that some maternal positions may worsen compression of the umbilical cord and decrease fetal blood flow. Maternal position changes may include left or right lateral, hands and knees, a high Fowlers with lateral tilt, or a slight Trendelenburg position. Further physiologic stress, such as supine hypotension, should be avoided to maximize uteroplacental blood flow. A fluid bolus often is administered in the presence of variable decelerations to increase intravascular blood volume and thereby optimize fetal oxygen perfusion. Such a bolus may require great caution or be contraindicated in cases of maternal cardiac disease and preeclampsia.

156

During the second stage, open glottal pushing or pushing with every other contraction may be helpful to minimize the severity of cord compression.

Amnioinfusion

Amnioinfusion performed according to hospital policies and protocols is an additional intervention that may be effective for decreasing significant variable and prolonged decelerations (Miyazaki & Navarez, 1985; Nageotte, Bertucci, Towers, Lagrew & Modlandou, 1991; Strong, 1995). Amnioinfusion is the instillation of fluid into the amniotic cavity to replace normal volumes of amniotic fluid lost with rupture of membranes or decreased volumes in situations of oligohydramnios. Amniotic fluid provides a cushioning effect for the fetus. The procedure uses an IUPC with a patent single or double lumen and an infusant similar to normal fetal electrolyte concentration, such as normal saline or lactated Ringer's solution. Protocols for instillation of fluid vary, but most recommend an initial bolus up to 800 ml, followed by a maintenance infusion to replace fluid that is lost (ACOG, 1995a). Further, some authorities recommend titration of the fluid bolus until decelerations are resolved, followed by an additional 250 ml (ACOG, 1995a; Miyazaki & Nevarez, 1985). If decelerations do not resolve, it may not be necessary to continue the infusion.

Amnioinfusion also may be used in the case of labor complicated by thick, particulate meconium. Thick, particulate meconium has been associated with an increased incidence of perinatal morbidity and mortality largely due to the risk of meconium aspiration syndrome (MAS). The use of amnioinfusion has been associated with decreased incidence of meconium found below the cords, increased fetal ability to tolerate labor, improved umbilical blood gases, reduction in cesarean births, and decreased need for operative intervention with lessened severity of variable decelerations (Dye, Aubry, Gross, & Artal, 1994; Erikson, Hostetter, & Parisi, 1994; Glantz & Letteney, 1996; Lameier & Katz, 1993; Macri et al., 1992; Strong, 1995; Uhing, Bhat, Philobus, & Raju, 1993).

It also has been suggested that amnioinfusion may decrease the incidence of postpartum endometritis in patients undergoing a cesarean delivery (Moen, Besinger, Tomich, & Fisher, 1995) and that the use of an antibiotic solution as an infusant may be beneficial in treating intramniotic infection (Strong, 1995; Paszkowski, 1994). Additional uses for antepartum abdominal amnioinfusion currently are being investigated. These include treatment of early oligohydramnios and infections, various diagnostic studies and treatment of failed versions in the late antepartum period (Lameier & Katz, 1993). However, further study is needed as inadequate data exist to draw conclusions about the effectiveness in these situations (Lameire & Katz, 1994; Strong, 1995).

Evaluation

When evaluating the effectiveness of amnioinfusion for significant variable or prolonged decelerations, it is important to consider that improvement in the fetal monitor tracing may require at least 20-30 minutes (ACOG, 1995a). If a tracing shows improvement with amnioinfusion, a reassuring fetal heart pattern is likely to continue. If the variable deceleration pattern does not improve despite an adequate bolus of infusant and replacement of lost fluid, or is accompanied by

157

decreased variability, interventions are continued and the physician or midwife are notified. The amnioinfusion may be discontinued in some cases while other interventions are continued. The woman's response to the procedure also is evaluated including uterine resting tone, contraction frequency and intensity, and the amount of fluid output (Wallerstedt, Higgins, Kasnic, & Curet, 1994).

Late Decelerations

Interventions for Late Decelerations

- Change to lateral position.
- Discontinue uterine stimulation.
- Increase fluid volume.
- Administer oxygen per mask.
- Consider tocolytic administration.
- Provide support and decrease anxiety.

The interventions that are provided to improve placental perfusion include changing the patient to a lateral position, which maximizes uteroplacental blood flow and avoids supine hypotension. Maximizing maternal fluid volume is thought to be beneficial to the fetus, as an increase in intravascular volume may correct hypotension as well as improve oxygen saturation to the fetus. Oxygen is more volume dependent than diffusion dependent. Therefore, a bolus of intravenous fluids may be an appropriate intervention unless contraindicated for medical reasons. Avoid dextrose IV fluids just prior to delivery if possible so that fetal hyperglycemia and rebound hypoglycemia are avoided.

If uterine stimulation by oxytocin or another uterine stimulant is being provided to the mother, its administration should be discontinued immediately if a late deceleration pattern is present. Other appropriate members of the health-care team (e.g., nurses, the primary provider, physicians/surgeons, midwife, anesthesiology personnel, neonatal care providers, and ancillary personnel) should be notified if assistance is needed.

Administration of oxygen to the mother may maximize oxygenation to the fetus by increasing maternal oxygen content. Oxygen is administered by a tight-fitting face mask to the mother, according to hospital protocol. The quantity may vary from 8-12 liters per minute depending upon the type of equipment used. Humidifying the oxygen during administration may increase maternal comfort. The administration of oxygen is maintained with decreased or absent variability. If the pattern is corrected and variability is present, the caregiver may discontinue the oxygen and observe the fetal response.

Tocolysis is used to provide uterine relaxation and to increase the uterine blood flow. It decreases or eliminates the reduction of uterine blood flow that occurs with uterine contraction.

The nurse and other caregivers have the responsibility to decrease patient anxiety, remain calm, provide clear directions to the patient as well as other members of the health-care team, and perform tasks confidently and competently. When explaining the situation to the patient, the caregiver should calmly, quickly, and factually state any concerns for the fetus, along with the need to provide interventions that may improve fetal status. During the time interventions are in progress, concise instructions and an explanation of events can be provided to the patient.

Evaluation

The correction of late decelerations implies that their etiology is a physiologic event that can be improved or corrected. However, when a late deceleration pattern persists despite corrective measures, other members of the health-care team should be summoned. If the pattern persists, variability is decreased, and/or the baseline becomes tachycardic as well, preparations for an expedient delivery should be initiated.

Early Decelerations

Interventions for Early Decelerations

No interventions are recommended for early decelerations, unless variability is absent or decreased, in which case the caregiver needs to reaffirm that the decelerations are early and not late decelerations. If the variability is absent or decreased, the caregiver needs to assess the fetal heart response to stimulation (scalp, abdominal, or vibroacoustic), reevaluate the management plan, and provide interventions as needed.

Prolonged Decelerations

Interventions for Prolonged Decelerations
- Change maternal position.
- Check for prolapsed cord or imminent delivery.
- Evaluate presenting part (rule out breech).
- Assess for identifiable cause, such as supine hypotension or sympathetic blockade secondary to regional anesthesia.
- Discontinue uterine stimulation.
- Give fluid bolus.
- Provide oxygen per mask.
- Provide tocolytics, as indicated.
- Perform amnioinfusion as ordered.
- Provide support and decrease anxiety.

The first interventions to improve the prolonged deceleration may include maternal position change. Assessing for identifiable causes may take place simultaneously with other interventions such as fluid bolus, oxygen, and/or decrease of uterine contractions by discontinuation of uterine stimulants (e.g., oxytocin or prostaglandin). Administration of a tocolytic, such as terbutaline, may be administered according to physician orders and hospital protocol. These actions may allow for intrauterine resuscitation.

When the nurse is the sole caregiver present, amnioinfusion may be a useful intervention that the nurse may provide under standardized procedures (if permitted by the state nurse practice act and hospital protocol). If successful, amnioinfusion may improve the fetal status. The nurse must act quickly and competently in such situations, and yet, at the same time, the nurse must provide patient instructions and explanations. A supportive and reassuring manner allays the patient's and support person's anxiety as rapid interventions are undertaken.

When a tocolytic is administered to a patient whose fetus is demonstrating a prolonged deceleration, the rapid decrease in uterine activity may decrease umbilical cord compression or improve uteroplacental blood flow and, therefore, improve fetal oxygenation. There is frequently an immediate improvement in the FHR.

If the deceleration cannot be corrected, immediate delivery may be necessary. Persistent prolonged decelerations may be caused by irreversible umbilical cord accidents, significant placental abruption, decreased blood flow to the fetus that cannot be corrected, or complications within the fetus itself.

Accelerations

Interventions for Accelerations

Nonperiodic accelerations observed as a response to sympathetic stimulation are indicative of a well-oxygenated CNS and no interventions are needed other than patient reassurance. In the presence of periodic accelerations or shoulders, possibly due to partial umbilical cord compression and fetal hypotension during contractions, altering maternal position may alter this pattern. Assessment of an accurate baseline rate is important when periodic accelerations are present (Freeman et al., 1991). The correct baseline may be perceived as decelerations if an incorrect assessment of baseline is perceived (Freeman et al., 1991). Regardless of whether accelerations are nonperiodic or periodic, the fetus is demonstrating a reassuring response.

In contrast, overshoot accelerations associated with variable decelerations necessitate repositioning, while observing variability. When variability is decreased, application of a spiral electrode will provide information regarding the fetal reserve. Hydration, oxygen administration, and notification of the physician or midwife is appropriate. The caregiver should reassure the patient and provide explanations for the interventions.

160

<u>Summary</u>

Decisions about interventions and use of further measures should be individualized in each patient situation, based on ongoing assessments. A decision-making tree that addresses the issues of intrapartum goals, physiologic interventions, and the use of additional measures/actions, such as instrumentation, is provided (Figure 4-4). This tree provides a general process outline which must be interpreted and modified, as appropriate, in light of the health care team's clinical assessment of the individual.

Decision Tree for Fetal Heart Monitoring

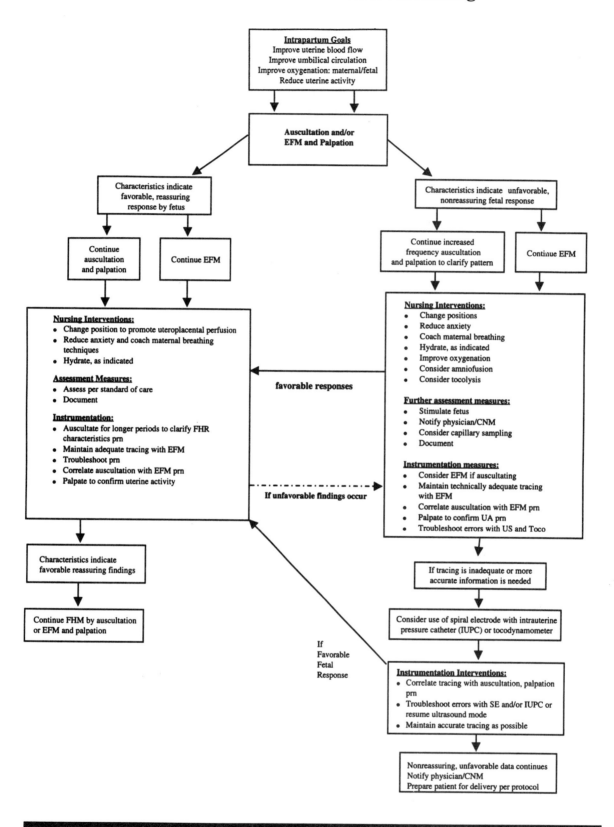

Figure 4-4. Decision tree for selection and verification of instrumentation techniques.

APPENDIX 4a: Technique of Fetal Scalp Sampling

The steps of fetal scalp sampling are provided in manuals, texts, as well as by manufacturers who produce disposable kits for sampling. Although the steps are simple, the actual sampling technique is a procedure that involves rupture of the membranes and requires experience. The equipment needed includes endoscope, light source, blade and bladeholder, sponges and holder, preheparinized capillary tubing, ethyl chloride, silicone grease, and blood gas analyzer. This procedure should be conducted only by a trained and qualified professional.

Principle Elements of Procedure

- Place patient in lateral position with top leg elevated (on raised side rail or held by assistant).
- Place the endoscope in the vagina and visualize scalp.
- Provide a light source.
- Clean scalp off with swabs.
- Spray with ethyl chloride to induce hyperemia (as per hospital protocol).
- Place silicone on skin to contain blood droplet.
- Perform a single or x-shaped puncture.
- Collect free-flowing blood in a heparinized glass tube.
- Mix blood using magnet and metal device in capillary tube.
- Collect two samples and then apply pressure to the area sampled with a sponge or swab until bleeding stops (at least through two uterine contractions).
- Test specimen per protocol. Record results on EFM tracing at the point the sample was obtained and in the designated section of the medical record (per hospital protocol).

APPENDIX 4b: Cord Blood Sampling at Time of Delivery

Sampling may be desired when the newborn status is compromised, is not compatible with intrapartum events, or reflects negatively on intrapartum events (see p. 151 for cord blood sampling indications). Obtaining cord blood samples will document the presence of acidosis, the type of acidosis, as well as provide information for resuscitation efforts and neonatal care.

Principal Elements of Procedure

- Obtain two 1 ml heparinized syringes for cord sampling.

- Attempt to have cord double-clamped prior to neonate's first breath.

- If cesarean delivery, request that a 6-8 inch segment of cord be double-clamped, cut, and passed off the surgical field to you as soon after the neonate is delivered as is possible.

- Draw samples from double-clamped cord segment within the hour. Put cord on a flat surface, straighten cord, palpate vessels, and insert needle into proper vessel. If drawing both a venous and arterial gas, draw from artery first.

- Aspirate 1 ml of blood from the umbilical artery, eliminate any blood in syringe, cap per protocol, and label specimen.

- Repeat same procedure for umbilical vein.

- To prevent inadvertently confusing specimens, pre-label syringes or place a smaller amount of blood in the arterial sample. (smaller vessel = smaller sample)

- Place on ice if specimen is not to be analyzed within the hour and transport to the laboratory.

- The specimen will remain stable at room temperature in a capped syringe for 30-60 minutes. (ACOG, 1995b).

APPENDIX 4c: Amnioinfusion

Amnioinfusion is a common procedure used to treat variable and prolonged decelerations during the first stage of labor and to dilute meconium below the vocal cords in labors complicated by thick, particulate meconium. It has been associated with a decreased need for operative interventions, improved cord gases, and an improved fetal heart tracing.

Principle Elements of Procedure

- The procedure requires rupture of membranes and placement of a single or double lumen IUPC.

- The hospital protocol should address the following issues:

    -- Contraindications to amnioinfusion.

    -- Who can perform amnioinfusion.

    -- What type of fluid may be used.

    -- Which instillation method is used—gravity flow and/or infusion pump.

    -- Which infusion techniques are used: bolus, continuous, or a combination of both.

    -- When and why the procedure is altered (e.g., loss of large amount of fluid due to position change or coughing, increased uterine resting tone, reappearance of abnormal FHR, or no uterine fluid return).

- Instill bolus at rate up to 800 ml or per hospital protocol.

- Maintain infusion at rate of 120-180 ml/hour (many authorities recommend to bolus until FHR improves and then add 250 ml) or per hospital protocol.

- Document purpose for procedure, fetal and maternal response to procedure, uterine resting tone, and amount of fluid output. The latter can be assessed by weighing pads or towels soaked with fluid.

- While warming the solution is no longer recommended for full-term fetuses, it may be appropriate for preterm or growth-restricted fetuses. Although rapid infusion of cold fluid causing bradycardia in a full-term fetus was reported in the literature (Miyazaki & Taylor, 1983), other studies have found no difference in outcomes when comparing the use of warmed versus room-temperature solutions (Glantz & Letteney, 1996; Nageotte, Bertucci, Towers, Lagrew, & Modlandou, 1991). Fluid, if warmed, should not be warmed in a microwave or blanket warmer as the temperature cannot be regulated and may result in injury to the fetus.

Nursing Considerations

- A lateral positioning is recommended during instillation.

- Benefits usually appear 20-30 minutes after infusion has begun (ACOG, 1995a).

- There have been case reports of polyhydramnios (Tabor & Maier, 1987), possible amniotic fluid embolism (Maher, Wenstrom, Hauth, & Meis, 1994), and cord prolapse. However, evidence is not conclusive that these risks are increased with use of amnioinfusion (Maher, Wenstrom, Hauth, & Meis, 1994). It remains appropriate to assess uterine resting tone and evaluate fluid output during amnioinfusion to avoid iatrogenic polyhydramnios (over distention of the uterus) during amnioinfusion. Polyhydramnios places the patient at risk for decreased uteroplacental perfusion, abruption with possible amniotic fluid embolism, and umbilical cord prolapse. Over distention may be more likely to occur when the fetal vertex obstructs outflow and may be corrected by withdrawal of even a small amount of fluid.

- If fetal bradycardia occurs when using a cold fluid infusion, discontinue the infusion and consider use of a blood warmer to warm the solution, or slow the infusion rate.

- Amnioinfusion appears to be safe in women undergoing a trial of labor after a previous cesarean section (Ouzounian, Miller, & Paul, 1996).

APPENDIX 4d: Vibroacoustic Stimulation

Vibroacoustic stimulation (VAS) is an additional method of fetal assessment. It has been used in the antepartum setting to decrease the incidence of false non-reactive stress tests (NST). Researchers have demonstrated that the use of VAS may decrease the testing time, lessen the probability of nonreactive NSTs, and decrease the need for retesting or using some other form of biophysical evaluation (Auyeung & Goldkrand, 1990; Miller-Slade et al., 1990; Sleutel, 1990).

While professional interpretation of its use during labor and its role in the intrapartum setting remains controversial, it is being examined as an alternative to fetal scalp sampling. In 1994, Smith found it to be as reliable as fetal scalp sampling for determining acidosis during the first stage of labor (Smith, 1994). Of those fetuses who responded to VAS with an acceleration exceeding 15 bpm for a 15 second duration, none were found to have an acidotic pH. Likewise, of the fetuses who did not respond to VAS, 53% had scalp pH < 7.20.

Principle Elements of Procedure

- The VAS procedure involves the use of a hand-held commercially distributed vibroacoustic stimulator and/or a battery-powered artificial larynx. This procedure should be performed according to established policies and protocol.

- The stimulus is applied over the fetal back or fetal head.

- Although the intensity of the stimulus may vary, it is usually between 80-110 dB. The duration of the stimulus should be at least 3 seconds, yet no greater than 5 seconds. If the fetus does not respond to the initial VAS, a second stimulation may be applied 3-10 minutes after the initial stimulus. If no response is achieved after the second VAS, further evaluation may be required (e.g., contraction stress test, oxytocin challenge test, or biophysical profile).

- Documentation should include a description of the tracing prior to VAS, the type of stimulus used, duration and position of stimulus applied, and the response to the stimulus by the fetus.

Nursing Considerations

Patient Education

- Explain the procedure and purpose to the patient.

- Demonstrate how the stimulus may feel on the maternal or nurse's forearm or leg, using firm but gentle pressure to apply the vibroacoustic stimulator against the skin. When the VAS device is used in open air, the sound may be louder and does not reflect the sound vibration level as accurately as when applied directly to the skin (Sleutel, 1990).

<u>Interpretation</u>

- Interpretation will depend on individual institutional guidelines. For example:
    - Reactive Vibroacoustic Stimulation Test (VST)
        - two accelerations, 15 bpm above the FHR baseline for > 15 seconds duration in a 10 minute period
    - Nonreactive VST
        - no accelerations in the allotted time
    - Equivocal VST
        - one acceleration meeting the stated criteria
        - accelerations not meeting the stated criteria
        - uninterpretable/unreadable fetal tracing

- The baseline FHR should be evaluated prior to stimulation. A tachycardic FHR may result from the stimulus and may last as long as one hour. If this should occur, observe for normal baseline characteristics other than the tachycardia. Observation of the fetus is continued until the FHR returns to the pre-stimulus range.

- The effect of gestational age on VST results is being explored. The incidence of reactive NSTs with the use of VAS may increase to as much as 89-100% in fetuses > 26 weeks of gestation (Smith, 1995). After 30 weeks of gestation, the effect of gestational age on fetal responses was found to be clinically insignificant (Gagnon, Benzaquen, & Hunse, 1992).

- The fetal response to VAS may be diminished or absent with the rupture of membranes and may decrease as labor progresses (Sleutel, 1989). There have been concerns about VAS resulting in prolonged FHR decelerations in pregnancies complicated by oligohydramnios. Sarno (1991) found that amniotic fluid volume was not related to the occurrence of prolonged decelerations.

<u>Safety</u>

Smith found that while prolonged exposure to sound levels of greater than 110 decibels could result in injury, it was unlikely to be harmful with a brief, non-repetitive stimulus (Smith, 1994). Arulkumaran and associates (1991) found no evidence of hearing loss in infants that received VAS in utero.

REFERENCES

ACOG Committee Opinion (1994). <u>Fetal distress and birth asphyxia</u> Washington, DC: Author.

ACOG Technical Bulletin (1995a). <u>Fetal heart rate patterns: Monitoring, interpretation, and management</u>. ACOG Technical Bulletin No. 207. Washington, DC: Author.

ACOG Technical Bulletin (1995b). <u>Umbilical artery blood acid-base analysis</u>. ACOG Technical Bulletin No. 216. Washington, DC: Author.

Arulkumaran, S., Skurr, B. A., Tong, H., Kek, L., K., & Ratnam, S. (1991). No evidence of hearing loss due to fetal acoustic stimulation test. <u>Obstetrics & Gynecology, 78</u>(2), 283-285.

Association of Women's Health, Obstetric and Neonatal Nurses (AWHONN). (1993). <u>Didactic content and clinical skills verification for professional nurse providers of basic, high risk, and critical care intrapartum nursing</u>. Washington, DC: Author.

Association of Women's Health, Obstetric and Neonatal Nurses (AWHONN). (1992). <u>Nursing responsibilities in implementing intrapartum fetal heart rate monitoring</u> (Position Statement). Washington, DC: Author.

Auyeung, R., & Goldkrand, J. (1990). Vibroacoustic stimulation and nursing intervention in the nonstress test. <u>Journal of Obstetric, Gynecologic, and Neonatal Nursing 20</u>(3), 232-238.

Cabaniss, M. (1993). <u>Fetal monitoring interpretation</u>. Philadelphia, PA: Lippincott-Raven Publication.

Cohen, W.R., & Schifrin, B.S. (1983). Diagnosis and management of the hypoxic fetal heart rate. In W.R. Cohen & E.A. Friedman (Eds.), <u>Management of labor.</u> Baltimore, MD: University Park Press.

Dye, T., Aubry, R., Gross, S., & Artal, R. (1994). Amnioinfusion and the intrauterine prevention of meconium aspiration. <u>American Journal of OB/GYN, 171,</u> 1601-1605.

Dickinson, J., Eriksen, N., Meyer, B., & Parisi, V. (1992). The effect of preterm birth on umbilical cord blood gases. <u>Obstetrics and Gynecology, 79,</u> 575-578.

Dildy, G.A., Clark, S.L., & Loucks, C.A. (1996). Intrapartum fetal pulse oximetry: Past, present, and future. <u>American Journal of Obstetrics and Gynecology, 175(1), 1-9.</u>

Duerbeck, N.B., Chaffin, D.G., & Seeds, J.W. (1992). A practical approach to umbilical artery pH and blood gas determinations. <u>Obstetrics and Gynecology, 79,</u> 959.

Erikson, N.L., Hostetter, M., & Parisi, V.M. (1994). Prophylactic amnioinfusion in pregnancies complicated by thick meconium. American Journal of Obstetrics and Gynecology, 171(4), 1026-30.

Fields, L.M., Entman, S.S., & Boehm, F.H. (1983). Correlation of the one minute Apgar score and the pH value of umbilical arterial blood. Southern Medical Journal, 76, 1477-1479.

Freeman, R.K., Garite, T.J., & Nageotte, M.D. (1991). Fetal heart rate monitoring (2nd ed.). Baltimore: Williams & Wilkins.

Gagnon, R., Benzaquen, S., & Hunse, C. (1992). The fetal sound environment during vibroacoustic stimulation in labor: Effect of fetal heart rate response. Obstetrics and Gynecology, 79(6), 950-955.

Gilstrap, L., Leveno, K., Burris, J., Williams, M., & Little, B. (1989). Diagnosis of birth asphyxia on the basis of fetal pH, Apgar score, and newborn cerebral dysfunction. American Journal of Obstetrics and Gynecology, 161, 825-830.

Gimovsky, M.L., & Caritis, S.N. (1982). Diagnosis and management of the hypoxic fetal heart rate. Clinics in Perinatology, 9(2), 313-324.

Glantz, J.C., & Letteney, D.L. (1996). Pumps and warmers during amnioinfusion: Is either necessary? Obstetrics & Gynecology, 87(1), 150-155.

Guyton A.C., (1992). Human physiology and mechanisms of disease (5th edition) Philadelphia, PA: W.B. Saunders Company.

Hon, E.H. (1975). An introduction to fetal heart rate monitoring (2nd ed.). Los Angeles: USC School of Medicine.

International Federation of Gynecology and Obstetrics (IFGO) Study Group on the Assessment of New Technology. (1995). Intrapartum surveillance: recommendations on current practice and overview of new developments.

Jauniaux, E., Jurkovic, D., Gulibis, B., Collins, W.P., Zaidi, J., & Campbell, S. (1994). Investigation of the acid-base balance of coelomic and amniotic fluids in early human pregnancy. American Journal of Obstetrics and Gynecology, 170(5), 1365-1369.

Lameier L., & Katz, V. (1993). Amnioinfusion: A review. Obstetrical and Gynecological Survey, 48, 829-837.

Macri, C., Schrimmer, D., Leung, A., Greenspoon, J., & Paul, R. (1992). Prophylactic amnioinfusion improves outcome of pregnancy complicated by thick meconium and oligohydramnios. American Journal of Obstetrics and Gynecology, 167, 117-121.

Martin, C. (1982). Physiology and clinical use of fetal heart rate variability. Clinics in Perinatology, 9(2), 339.

Miller-Slade, D., Gloeb, D., Bailey, S., Bendell, A., Interlandi, E., Kline-Kaye, V., & Kroesen, J. (1990). Acoustic stimulation-induced fetal response compared to traditional nonstress testing. Journal of Obstetric, Gynecologic, and Neonatal Nursing, 20(2), 160-167.

Miyazaki, F.S., & Nevarez, F. (1985). Saline amnioinfusion for relief of repetitive variable decelerations: A prospective randomized study. American Journal of Obstetrics and Gynecology, 153, 301-306.

Moen, M. D., Besinger, R. E., Tomich, P. G., & Fisher, S.G. (1995). Effect of amnioinfusion on the incidence of postpartum endometritis in patients undergoing cesarean delivery. Journal of Reproductive Medicine, 40, 383-386.

Moll, W., & Kastendieck, E. (1985). Kinetics of lactic acid accumulation and removal in the fetus. In W. Kunzel (Ed.), Fetal heart rate monitoring. Clinical practice and pathophysiology. Berlin: Springer-Verlag.

Murray, M. (1988). Antepartal and intrapartal fetal monitoring. Washington, DC: NAACOG.

Murray, M. (1996). Antepartal and intrapartal fetal monitoring, (2nd ed.). Albuquerque, NM: Learning Resources International, Inc.

Nageotte, M.P., Bertucci, L., Towers, G., Lagrew, P.L., & Modanlov, H. (1991). Prophylactic amnioinfusion in pregnancies complicated by oligohydramnius. Obstetrics & Gynecology, 77(5), 677-680

Newman, W., Mitchell, P., & Wood, C. (1967). Fetal acid-base status II. Relationship between maternal and fetal blood bicarbonate concentrations. American Journal of Obstetrics and Gynecology, 97(1), 52-57.

Nurses Association of the American College of Obstetricians and Gynecologists (NAACOG). (1991). Nursing practice competencies and educational guidelines: Antepartum fetal surveillance and intrapartum fetal heart monitoring. Washington, DC: Author.

Ouzounian, J. G., Miller, D. A., & Paul, R. H. (1996). Amnioinfusion in women with previous cesarean births: A preliminary report. American Journal of Obstetrics & Gynecology, 174, 783-786.

Parer, J.T. (1989). Fetal heart rate. In R.K. Creasy & R. Resnik (Eds.), Maternal fetal medicine: Principles and practice (p. 314). Philadelphia: W.B. Saunders.

Parer, J.T. (1997). Handbook of fetal heart rate monitoring, 2nd Ed. Philadelphia: W.B. Saunders Company.

Paszkowski, T. (1994). Amnioinfusion: A review. Journal of Reproductive Medicine, 39, 588-594.

Petrie, R. (1991). Intrapartum fetal evaluation. In S. Gabbe, J. Niebyl, & J. Simpson, Obstetrics: Normal and problem pregnancies (2nd ed.) (p. 457). New York: Churchill Livingstone.

Phelan, J., Ahn, M., Korst, L., & Martin, G. (1995). Nucleated red blood cells: A marker for fetal asphyxia? American Journal of OB/GYN, 173, 1380-1384.

Simpson, K., & Creehan, P. (1996). Perinatal nursing. Philadelphia, PA: Lippincott - Raven Publication.

Sleutel, M. (1989). An overview of vibroacoustic stimulation. Journal of Obstetric, Gynecologic, and Neonatal Nursing, Nov/Dec, 447-452.

Sleutel, M. (1990). Vibroacoustic stimulation and fetal heart rate in nonstress test. Journal of Obstetric, Gynecologic, and Neonatal Nursing, 19(3), 199-204.

Smith, C. (1994). Vibroacoustic stimulation for risk assessment. Clinics in Perinatology, 21(4), 797-808.

Smith C. (1995). Vibroacoustic stimulation. Clinical Obstetrics and Gynecology, 38(1), 68-77.

Society of Obstetricians and Gynaecologists of Canada (SOGC). (1995). SOGC Policy Statement: Fetal health surveillance in labour. Journal of SOGC, 17(9), 865-901.

Sonek. J., & Nicolaides, K. (1994). The role of cordocentesis in the diagnosis of fetal well-being. Clinics in Perinatology, 21(4), 743-764.

Strong, T. H. (1995). Amnioinfusion. Journal of Reproductive Medicine, 40(2), 108-114.

Sykes, G., Johnson, E., & Ashworth, F. (1982). Do Apgar scores indicate asphyxia? Lancet, 1, 494.

Uhing, M. R., Bhat, R., Philobus, M., & Raju, T.N.K. (1993). Value of amnioinfusion in reducing meconium aspiration syndrome. American Journal of Perinatology, 10, 43-45.

Wallerstedt, C., Higgins, P., Kasnic, T., & Curet, L. (1994). Amnioinfusion: An update. Journal of Obstetric, Gynecologic, and Neonatal Nursing, 23, 573-578.

Wenstrom, K., Andrews, W.W., & Maher, J. E. (1995). Amnioinfusion survey: Prevalence, protocols, and complications. Obstetrics & Gynecology, 86(4.1), 572-576.

Winkler, D., Hauth, J., Tucker, J., Owen, J., & Brumfield, C. (1991). Neonatal complications at term as related to the degree of umbilical artery acidemia. American Journal of Obstetrics and Gynecology, 164, 637-641.

Yeomans, E. R., Hauth, J. C., Gilstrap, L. C., & Strickland, D. M. (1985). Umbilical cord pH, PCO_2, and bicarbonate following uncomplicated term vaginal deliveries. American Journal of Obstetrics and Gynecology, 151, 798-900.

BIBLIOGRAPHY

American Academy of Pediatrics and American College of Obstetricians and Gynecologists (AAP & ACOG). (1992). Guidelines for Perinatal Care (3rd ed.). Elk Grove Village, IL: Author.

Arbitol, M. M. (1985). Supine position in labor and associated fetal heart rate changes. Obstetrics and Gynecology, 65, 481-486.

Barnett, W.M. (1989). Umbilical cord prolapse: A true obstetrical emergency. Journal of Emergency Medicine, 7(2), 149-152.

Baxi, L. V. (1982). Current status of fetal oxygen monitoring. Clinics in Perinatology, 9, 423-430.

Beall, M. H., Edgar, B. W., Paul, R., & Smith-Wallace, T. (1985). A comparison of ritodrine, terbutaline, and magnesium sulfate for the suppression of term labor. American Journal of Obstetrics and Gynecology, 153, 854-858.

Boehm, F. H. (1990). Fetal distress. In R. D. Eden & F. H. Boehm (Eds.), Assessment and care of the fetus. Norwalk, CT: Appleton and Lange.

Burke, M. S., Porreco, R. P., Day, D., Watson, J. D., Haverkamp, A. D., Orleans, M., & Luckey, D. (1989). Intrauterine resuscitation with tocolysis. An alternate month clinical trial. Journal of Perinatology, 9, 296-300.

Caldeyro-Barcia, R. (1979). The influence of maternal bearing-down efforts during second stage on fetal well-being. Birth and the Family Journal, 6(1), 17-21.

Campbell, W. A., Vintzileos, A. M., & Nochimson, D. J. (1986). Intrauterine versus extrauterine management/resuscitation of the fetus/neonate. Clinical Obstetrics and Gynecology, 29, 33-42.

Chauhan, S. P. (1990). Does prophylactic amnioinfusion make a difference? (Letter). American Journal of Obstetrics and Gynecology, 163, 1370-1371.

Cohen, W. R. (1977). Influence of the duration of second stage labor on perinatal outcome and puerperal morbidity. Obstetrics and Gynecology, 49, 266.

Crino, J.P., Harris, A.P., Parisi, V.M., & Johnson, T.R.B. (1993). Effects of rapid intravenous crystalloid infusion on uteroplacental blood flow and placental implantation-site oxygen delivery in the pregnant ewe. American Journal of Obstetrics and Gynecology, 168(5), 1603-1609.

Fisk, N. M., Tannirandorn, Y., Nicolin, U., Talbert, D. G., & Rodeck, C. H. (1990). Amniotic pressure in disorders of amniotic fluid volume. Obstetrics and Gynecology, 76, 210-214.

173

Galvan, B. J., Van Mullem, C., & Broekhuizen, F. F. (1989). Using amnioinfusion for the relief of repetitive variable decelerations during labor. Journal of Obstetric, Gynecologic, and Neonatal Nursing, 15, 222-229.

Garite, T. J. (1990). Premature rupture of the membranes. In R. D. Eden & F. H. Boehm (Eds.), Assessment and care of the fetus. Norwalk, CT: Appleton and Lange.

Goldaber, K., Gilstrap, L., Leveno, K., Dax, J., & McIntire, D. (1991). Pathologic fetal acidemia. Obstetrics and Gynecology, 78, 1103-1107.

Goodlin, R. C. (1986). Mechanism of amnioinfusion (Letter). American Journal of Obstetrics and Gynecology, 155, 1359-1360.

Goodlin, R. C. (1989). The prevention of meconium aspiration in labor using amnioinfusion (Letter). Obstetrics and Gynecology, 74, 430-431.

Goodlin, R. C. (1991). Was there really a difference with amnioinfusion? (Letter). American Journal of Obstetrics and Gynecology, 164, 235-236.

Goodlin, R. C., & Ingram, M. (1990). Ultrasonic study of amnioinfusion. A report of two cases. Journal of Reproductive Medicine, 35, 439-440.

Griese, M.E., & Prickett, S.A. (1993). Nursing management of umbilical cord prolapse. Journal of Obstetric, Gynecologic, and Neonatal Nursing, 22(4), 311-315.

Harvey, C., & Chez, B. F. (1996). Critical concepts in fetal heart rate monitoring (2nd ed.). Videotape series: Association of Women's Health, Obstetric and Neonatal Nurses. Baltimore, MD: Williams and Wilkins.

Haubrich, K. L. (1990). Amnioinfusion: A technique for the relief of variable deceleration. Journal of Obstetric, Gynecologic, and Neonatal Nursing, 19, 299-303.

Huddleston, J. F. (1984). Management of acute fetal distress in the intrapartum period. Clinical Obstetrics and Gynecology, 27, 84-94.

Huddleston, J. F. (1990). Electronic fetal monitoring. In R. D. Eden & F. H. Boehm (Eds.), Assessment and care of the fetus. Norwalk, CT: Appleton and Lange.

Hutson, J. M., & Mueller-Heubach, E. (1982). Diagnosis and management of intrapartum reflex fetal heart rate changes. Clinics in Perinatology, 9, 325-337.

Imanaka, M., Ogita, S., & Sugawa, T. (1989). Saline solution amnioinfusion for oligohydramnios after premature rupture of membranes: A preliminary report. American Journal of Obstetrics and Gynecology, 161, 102-106.

174

Ingemarrson, I., Arulkumaran, S., & Ratnam, S. S. (1985). Single injection of terbutaline in term labor: I. Effect on fetal pH cases with prolonged bradycardia. American Journal of Obstetrics and Gynecology, 153, 859-864.

Ingemarrson, I., Arulkumaran, S., & Ratnam, S. S. (1985). Single injection of terbutaline in term labor: II. Effect on uterine activity. American Journal of Obstetrics and Gynecology, 153, 865-869.

Jacobs, M. M., & Phibbs, R. H. (1989). Prevention, recognition and treatment of perinatal asphyxia. Clinics in Perinatology, 16, 785-807.

Katz, Z., Shoham (Schwartz), Z., Lancet, M., Blickstien, I., Mogilner, B.M., & Zalel, Y. (1988). Management of labor with umbilical cord prolapse: A 5-year study. Obstetrics and Gynecology, 72(2), 278-281.

Khan, S., Ahmed, G., Abutaleb, A., & Hathal, M. (1995). Is the determination of umbilical cord arterial blood gases necessary in all deliveries? Analysis of a high risk population. Journal of Perinatalogy, 15, 39-42.

Kilbride, K. W., Yeast, J. D., & Thibeault, D. W. (1989). Intrapartum and delivery room management of premature rupture of membranes complicated by oligohydramnios. Clinics in Perinatology, 16, 863-888.

Knorr, L.J. (1989). Relieving fetal distress with amnioinfusion. Maternal Child Nursing, 14, 346-350.

Lee, W., & Cotton, D. B. (1990). Maternal cardiovascular physiology. In R. D. Eden & F. H. Boehm (Eds.), Assessment and care of the fetus. Norwalk, CT: Appleton and Lange.

Levy, J., & Rosenzweig, B. (1986). Amnioinfusion for fetal distress (Letter). American Journal of Obstetrics and Gynecology, 155, 1361.

Lipshitz, J., Shaver, D. C., & Anderson, O. D. (1986). Hexoprenaline tocolysis for intrapartum fetal distress and acidosis. Journal of Reproductive Medicine, 31, 1023-1026.

Mandruzzato, G., Meir, Y.J., & Gigli, C. (1994). Fetal blood sampling in labor. Journal of Perinatal Medicine, 22, 485-489.

McKay, S. (1984). Squatting: An alternate position for the second stage of labor. Maternal Child Nursing, 9, 181-183.

McKay, S., & Roberts, J. (1985). Second stage labor: What is normal? Journal of Obstetric, Gynecologic, and Neonatal Nursing, 14, 101-106.

Miller, F. C. (1981). Quantitation of uterine activity. Clinics in Perinatology, 8, 27-34.

Miyazaki, F., & Taylor, N. (1983). Saline amnioinfusion for relief of variable or prolonged decelerations. <u>American Journal of Obstetrics and Gynecology, 14,</u> 670.

Miyazaki, F., & Nevarez, F. (1985). Saline amnioinfusion for relief of repetitive variable decelerations: A prospective randomized study. <u>American Journal of Obstetrics and Gynecology, 153,</u> 301.

Nageotte, M. P. (1987). Reversible antepartum fetal distress. <u>Clinical Obstetrics and Gynecology, 30,</u> 999-1006.

Noble, E. (1981). Controversies in maternal effort during labor and delivery. <u>Journal of Nurse-Midwifery, 26,</u> 13-22.

Nyman, M., Arulkumaran, S., Jakobsson, J., & Westgren, M. (1992). Vibro-acoustic stimulation in high-risk pregnancies: Maternal perception of fetal movement, fetal heart rate and fetal outcome. <u>Journal of Perinatal Medicine, 20,</u> 267-274.

Owen, J., Henson, B. V., & Hauth, J. C. (1990). <u>American Journal of Obstetrics and Gynecology, 162,</u> 1146-1149.

Patriarco, M. S., Viechnicki, B. M., Hutchinson, T. A., Klasko, S. K., & Yeh, S. (1987). A study on intrauterine fetal resuscitation with terbutaline. <u>American Journal of Obstetrics and Gynecology, 157,</u> 384-387.

Petrie, R. H. (1981). The pharmacology and use of oxytocin. <u>Clinics in Perinatology, 8,</u> 35-47.

Phelan, J. P., Stine, L. G., Mueller, E., McCart, D., & Yeh, S. (1984). Observations of fetal heart rate characteristics related to cephalic version and tocolysis. <u>American Journal of Obstetrics and Gynecology, 149,</u> 658-661.

Piquard, F., Hsiung, J. R., Mettauer, M., Schaefer, A., Haberey, P., & Dellenbach, P. (1988). The validity of fetal heart rate monitoring during the second stage of labor. <u>Obstetrics and Gynecology, 72,</u> 746-751.

Posner, M. D., Ballagh, S. A., & Paul, R. H. (1990). The effect of amnioinfusion on uterine pressure and activity: A preliminary report. <u>American Journal of Obstetrics and Gynecology, 163,</u> 813-818.

Resnik, R., & Gilbert, W. M. (1990). Myometrial physiology. In R. D. Eden & F.H. Boehm (Eds.), <u>Assessment and care of the fetus.</u> Norwalk, CT: Appleton and Lange.

Roberts, J. E. (1989). Managing fetal bradycardia during second stage of labor. <u>Maternal Child Nursing, 14,</u> 394-398.

Roberts, J. E., Gruener, J. S., & Mendez-Bauer, C. (1987). A descriptive analysis of involuntary bearing-down efforts during the expulsive phase of labor. Journal of Obstetric, Gynecologic, and Neonatal Nursing, 16, 48.

Sadovosky, Y., Amon, E., Bade, M. E., & Petrie, R. H. (1989). Prophylactic amnioinfusion during labor complicated by meconium: A preliminary report. American Journal of Obstetrics and Gynecology, 161, 613-618.

Sala, D. J., & Moise, K. J. (1990). The treatment of preterm labor using a portable subcutaneous terbutaline pump. Journal of Obstetric, Gynecologic, and Neonatal Nursing, 19, 108-115.

Schmidt, S. (1988). Methodology and clinical value of transcutaneous blood gas measurements in the fetus. Journal of Perinatal Medicine, 16(Suppl. 1), 95-105.

Shalev, E., Blondheim, O., & Peleg, D. (1995). Use of cordocentesis in the management of preterm or growth restricted fetuses with abnormal monitoring. Obstetrical and Gynecological Survey, 50, 839-844.

Steiger, R. M., & Nageotte, M. P. (1990). Effect of uterine contractility and maternal hypotension on prolonged decelerations after bupivacaine epidural anesthesia. American Journal of Obstetrics and Gynecology, 163, 808-812.

Stookey, R. A., Sokol, R. J., & Rosen, M. G. (1973). Abnormal contraction patterns in patients monitored during labor. Obstetrics and Gynecology, 42, 359.

Strickland, D., Gilstrap, L., Hauth, J., & Widmer, K. (1984). Umbilical cord pH and PCO_2: Effect of interval from delivery to determination. American Journal of Obstetrics and Gynecology, 148, 191-194.

Strong, T. H., Hetzler, G., Sarno, A. P., & Paul, R. H. (1990). Prophylactic intrapartum amnioinfusion: A randomized clinical trial. American Journal of Obstetrics and Gynecology, 162, 1370-1374.

Wenstrom, K., & Parsons, M. (1989). Prevention of meconium aspiration in labor using amnioinfusion. Obstetrics & Gynecology, 73,(4) 647-651.

Willcourt, R., & Queenan, J. T. (1981). Fetal scalp blood sampling and transcutaneous PO_2. Clinics in Perinatology, 8, 87-99.

Yeoman, E., Hauth, J., Gilstrap, L., & Strickland, D. (1985). Umbilical cord pH, PCO_2, and decarbonate following uncomplicated term vaginal deliveries. American Journal of Obstetrics and Gynecology, 151, 798-800.

Young, B. (1990). Placental regulation of fetal oxygenation and acid-base balance. In R. D. Eden & F. H. Boehm (Eds.), Assessment and care of the fetus. Norwalk, CT: Appleton and Lange.

CHAPTER 5: EVALUATION

Ongoing critical decision-making requires evaluation. Evaluation of the maternal-fetal status provides feedback for each phase of the nursing process (Figure 5-1). Outcomes are used to determine whether initial assessments, interpretations, diagnoses, and interventions were appropriate and effective. An evaluation algorithm is presented (Figure 5-2). Evaluation is a thread that links together each part of the problem-solving approach (Figure 5-1).

Interventions in this chapter refer to those interventions used specifically to promote four intrapartum physiologic goals. These four primary goals are promoting uterine blood flow, umbilical circulation, oxygenation (maternal/fetal), and normal uterine activity. Management is a more comprehensive term that includes interventions to promote these goals as well as additional assessments and actions that may have a direct or indirect effect on the maternal-fetal status. It is important to view the fetal monitoring data in light of the entire clinical picture. Management includes independent and collaborative assessments and actions.

Evaluation of maternal-fetal responses to specific interventions and overall management includes ongoing systematic reviews of current fetal heart characteristics and uterine activity. The trends in the fetal heart data within the context of the current maternal-fetal status need to be examined. It is important to consider whether the assessments and interpretations of the fetal heart monitoring data have changed. A re-evaluation of whether the collaborative problems initially identified remain pertinent is useful (Figure 5-2). The method of monitoring may need to be changed on the basis of the evaluations made. The reader is referred to the Decision Tree for Fetal heart Monitoring (Figure 2-21) in Chapter 2, for a review of selection and verification of instrumentation techniques.

Evaluation must take into consideration maternal responses because an intervention may alter the maternal condition, which in turn may affect the fetus. In addition to reassessing the fetal heart monitoring data, it is important to reconsider other ongoing maternal-fetal assessments. Examples of additional maternal assessments include maternal-fetal history, changes in risk factors, any medications administered, maternal vital sign changes, and other individual factors that may affect the maternal-fetal status.

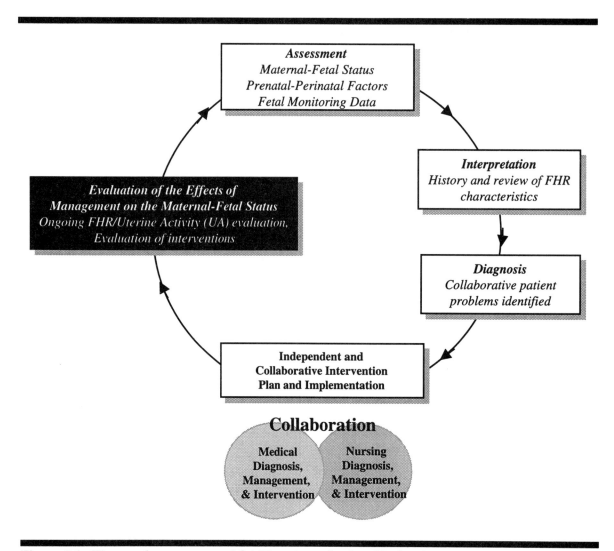

Figure 5-1. The nursing process and fetal heart monitoring: Evaluation

Evaluation in fetal monitoring involves making one or more decisions about what further action(s) to take. Three basic options exist:

1.   Discontinue intervention(s)
   • Problem resolved
   • Negative physiologic influence eliminated

2.   Alter intervention(s)
   • New or additional physiologic factors may have occurred
   • Initial interpretations may not be validated or may have changed

3.   Continue current intervention(s)
   • The original physiologic factors which required intervention remain (Figure 5-2).

In summary, on-going evaluation of the assessment, interpretations, diagnoses, and interventions implemented are important elements of the evaluation of the effects of management on the maternal fetal-status. Determining whether the desired changes in the fetal response have occurred is a primary focus of the evaluation process. Although the focus of evaluation here is on the response of the fetus to physiologic interventions, ongoing evaluation also includes a review of the nurse's communication with the patient, significant others, and other health care providers. Further discussion of communication principles continues in Chapter 6.

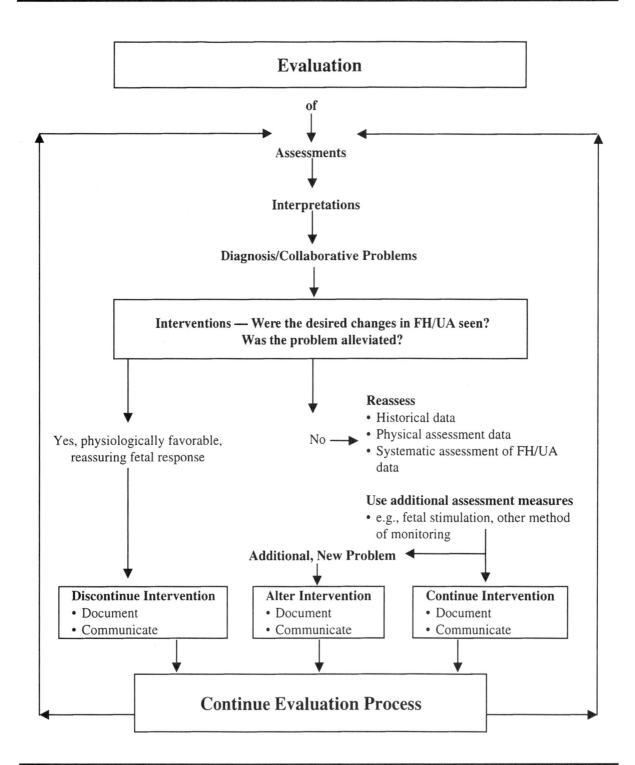

Figure 5-2. Decision-making process for evaluation of the effectiveness of management and intervention outcomes.

CHAPTER 6: COMMUNICATION

Introduction

Communication is a thread that links each step of the nursing process (Figure 6-1). Communication may be verbal, nonverbal, or written and includes the ability to listen. This chapter outlines principles for communication, conflict resolution, and documentation.

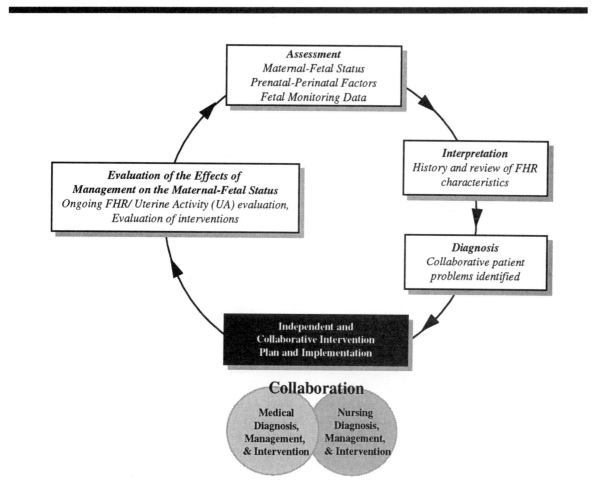

Figure 6-1. The nursing process and fetal heart monitoring: Communication

183

Purpose and Significance

Interprofessional communication, between nurses or between the nurse and the physician or mid-wife, has important implications for patient care from both medical and legal perspectives (NAACOG, 1987c).

Communication should focus on the benefit of the patient. Therefore, nurse-physician/midwife interactions, as well as nurse-nurse interactions, should be directed toward meeting patient needs. Interactions should focus on assessment, observations, and requests about patient care (NAACOG, 1987c), as well as report any change in the status of the mother or fetus. Verbal communication also includes the professional responsibility of the nurse to keep the patient informed about her care and treatment. Finally, the nurse needs to listen to the patient. Active listening can dispel patient fear and increase a patient's level of trust. Experts agree that a decreased likelihood of malpractice litigation appears to exist when effective communication occurs.

An important component of communication between professionals is education. Comprehensive orientation programs and ongoing planned educational classes help nurses update both the knowledge and skills associated with fetal heart monitoring. Orientation programs should include didactic content and directed clinical supervision to ensure the competence of nurses in applying the monitoring equipment, interpreting tracings, reporting and documenting events, implementing communication policies, and meeting expectations as a member of a health care team. (NAACOG, 1991).

Method of Communication

Communication is multifaceted and involves verbal, nonverbal, written, computer, and telecommunications channels. Communication also is multidirectional in its transmission and reception. The following examples illustrate how these characteristics of communications affect health care and fetal heart monitoring (FHM).

Nurse-to-Nurse Communication

As shifts change and a different group of nurses arrives to care for patients, a reporting mechanism is used to ensure continuity of care. Short-term reports for continuity of care occur when nurses relieve each other for breaks or when patient assignments are altered during shifts. During the antepartum and intrapartum phase, the content of these reports includes FHR and FHM events and status.

FHM information transmitted from nurse-to-nurse highlights not only what is heard or observed of the fetal heart, but also events that potentially influence the FHR and patterns. Events influencing the fetal heart are many and include gravidity, parity, gestational age, maternal health and habits, maternal intake of medications, cervical status (effacement, dilatation), station, and status of membranes. If the membranes are ruptured, the time of rupture and character of the amniotic fluid are important assessments. The progress of labor, uterine contractions (frequency, duration, intensity, and resting tone), hydration, analgesia, and anesthesia may affect the quality of uteroplacental blood flow, fetal status, and fetal heart characteristics.

The effectiveness of nurse-to-nurse communication potentially influences continuity of maternal-fetal care, and thus, fetal status and well-being. Examples of effective communication include information that is shared regarding the results of previous interventions to improve fetal heart status, patient responses to labor, and location of the physician for rapid accessibility if needed.

<u>Nurse-to-Nurse Communication Related to FHM</u>

- Occurs at shift report.
- Occurs anytime care is transferred to another nurse.
- Occurs when maternal or fetal status changes.

All of the above are dynamic occurrences, especially during the intrapartum period, and require ongoing communication between nurses.

Nurse-to-Primary Care Provider Communication

Nurse-to-primary care provider (physician, midwife) communication focuses on maternal-fetal needs and, in FHM, upon the interpretation of fetal heart data. Many of the features of nurse-to-nurse communication previously described also are present in nurse-to-physician/midwife communication.

The nurse has the responsibility of informing the physician/midwife of changes in maternal or fetal status. This necessitates providing clear, descriptive information to assist the physician/midwife in making a medical judgement, communicating specific requests (e.g., the physician's or midwife's presence or analgesia for the woman), and presenting the information in a timely manner. When the primary care provider is not immediately present, the nurse-to-physician/midwife conversation often occurs via telephone, often with the assistance of other electronic media such as a facsimile, telecopier, or computer terminal. Sharing written information (e.g., copy of the tracing) with the provider may be helpful in some situations to clarify the verbal communication.

<u>Nurse-to-Primary Care Provider Communication Related to FHM</u>

- Communicate information that concerns fetal heart status.
- Report clearly, concisely, comprehensively, and in a timely manner.
- Make requests direct and clear.

Nurse-to-Patient Communication

Both the physician or midwife and the nurse have a duty to ensure that the patient is informed of care and treatment information, including fetal heart monitoring data. While informed consent is the physician's or midwife's responsibility, the nurse assesses patient understanding of explanations regarding the care. The nurse assumes responsibility for discussing the nursing plan of care with the mother.

The nurse is aware that "informed consent is a process of education and discussion. The heart of informed consent is the explanation to the patient of the proposed treatment so that she can make an informed consent or refusal of care. The patient is informed about the method of monitoring based on

185

institution policy and collaborative decision making between patient, physician, and nurse" (NAACOG, 1987b).

The nurse continually provides the patient with information regarding maternal as well as fetal status. Providing information about care, treatment, status, and impending events during the flow of nurse-to-patient conversation assists in achieving a positive outcome. Listening to patient requests, concerns, and needs; responding appropriately; and providing the above information in a manner that reduces anxiety and enhances patient participation is also important. It has been shown that there is a correlation between the continuous presence of a trained support person and less negative ratings of women's childbirth experiences and less maternal tenseness (Enkin, Keirse, Renfrew, & Nelson, 1995). In addition, the presence of a trained person was associated with other positive clinical outcomes including decreased likelihood of pain, decreased incidence of operative vaginal deliveries, and fewer cesarean births (Enkin et al., 1995).

Nurse-to-Patient Communication Related to FHM

- Explain ongoing care and treatment according to hospital policy.
- Inform patient of maternal and fetal status, as needed.
- Reduce anxiety, enhance participation.
- Listen and respond to patient requests.

Conflict Resolution

Circumstances can occur in which there will be conflict about the plan of care. The overall goal of involved parties is to provide quality care and promote optimal outcomes for both mother and newborn. Maintaining mutual respect among the various professional disciplines providing care in the perinatal setting is important. It is important when a conflict occurs to keep sight of these basic ideals (Simpson & Chez, 1996).

Conflict can be referred to as "the internal discord that results from differences in ideas, values, or feelings of two or more people" (with Marquis & Huston, 1992, p. 312). Conflict in any setting is a natural occurrence. It is important to acknowledge that conflict exists. The outcome of conflict may be either positive or negative depending on how the conflict is managed. Ideally, the goal of creating a win-win situation for all parties involved is desirable. When parties involved in a conflict are able to identify and work toward a common goal, the result is collaboration (Marquis & Huston, 1992). This may not always be possible. Strategies used to resolve conflict are affected by the issues in the conflict situation, the degree of urgency involved, and individuals involved in the conflict.

The ability to communicate, to focus on treatment versus personal issues, and to identify and focus on a common goal are factors that may positively affect conflict resolution outcomes (Marquis & Huston, 1992; Simpson & Chez, 1996). It is important to avoid tactics, such as using ridicule, implying guilt, using aggression, or conversely, avoiding action (Marquis & Huston, 1992). It also is important to develop strategies to deal with these tactics when they are being used in negotiation to resolve conflict.

Strategies that may improve communication include the following: use statements based on research, listen actively and observe the nonverbal cues, maintain an open mind to establish a cooperative environment, try to understand the other person's perspective, discuss the conflict (not personal issues), avoid attaching blame, be honest, know what your limits are and "what the bottom line" is, and take a break when emotions take over as time allows (Marquis & Huston, 1992). An additional strategy is to identify areas or goals where agreement exists.

There is a time and a place for discussion. In perinatal health care settings, it is desirable to resolve the conflict outside the presence of the woman and her family, visitors, and other non-involved parties. It is important to address conflict situations and to seek closure after the conflict has been addressed. Ideally, similar conflicts may be avoided in the future.

Conflict can occur in a perinatal setting when

- A new or alternate plan of care is presented.
- There is a difference of opinion over the management of a patient.

When time permits, the most successful means of resolving a conflict include

- Using a calm approach and taking the time to listen to all opinions.
- Avoiding body language that signals hostility.
- Selecting an appropriate venue, away from patients, the public, and uninvolved colleagues.
- Providing a reasonable rationale for the plan of care.
- Stating each perspective in terms of "I" and taking responsibility for that perspective. For example, "I am confused, I thought our plan of care was based on . . . " or "I am not reassured by this fetal response for the following reasons . . . "
- Avoiding comments that blame or are critical of the other person, such as, "You are wrong." Instead, ask the person to explain their perspective. For example, "Please tell me more about what you see in this situation that is reassuring about the fetal status . . . " or "Help me understand your perspective . . . "
- Keeping the conversation directed toward patient care and possible impact on outcome.
- Involving an objective third person, as needed, can keep the situation from becoming confrontational.
- Avoiding and not tolerating verbal abuse.
- Postponing the discussion to help calm involved parties when time and circumstances allow.

(Marquis & Huston, 1992; Simpson & Chez, 1996)

Most situations can be resolved by addressing concerns quickly and providing as clear and complete a picture of the details as possible. Inappropriate decisions often are based on incomplete information.

Chain of Command

When the potential exists for rapid deterioration of the maternal and/or fetal condition, and discussions with the physician or midwife have not led to an agreement of appropriate care within a particular clinical situation, the primary nurse may need to initiate the "chain-of-command." The protocol for use of the "chain of command" is usually outlined in the policy and procedure manual for each institution or perinatal setting. In some clinical practice settings, this also may be referred to as the "chain of consultation" (SOGC, 1995, p. 39). It is beneficial to know the procedure before a situation occurs. State or Province Nurse Practice Acts also address nursing accountability (e.g., "the nurse is a patient advocate . . . "). It is important to know what each jurisdiction's Nurse Practice Act requires with regard to this issue. Failure to use chain of command in situations of extreme conflict and/or emergency may increase the likelihood of adverse patient outcome and nursing liability if the situation later results in litigation. Figures 6-2, 6-3 and 6-4 provide examples of chain-of command.

Every perinatal care setting should have a written protocol for chain of command to ensure optimal and timely management of patients when a conflict or problem exists (Figure 6-2). The interaction of professional communication can be summarized in a flowchart showing possible accountabilities. This format is merely a suggestion, and alternate plans are possible, depending on the clinical setting or policy of the institution. In an emergency situation the chain of command initially includes going to the next level of authority. However in the best interest of the patient, movement though the chain may occur more rapidly and the person(s) contacted may vary depending on the nature of the clinical circumstances and the time available. Some alternate examples of chain of command involving different professionals are explored in Figures 6-3 and 6-4. In any of the possible scenarios, it is important to make clear to the parties involved that the chain of command is being initiated when all other attempts to resolve the conflict have not resulted in appropriate care.

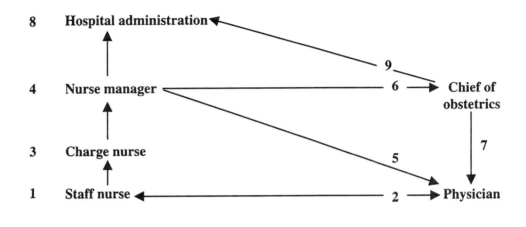

Figure 6-2. Example of problem resolution relying on chain of command (Chez, Harvey, & Murray, 1990).

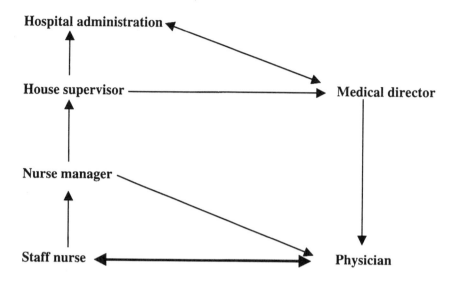

Figure 6-3. Example of problem resolution relying on chain of command.

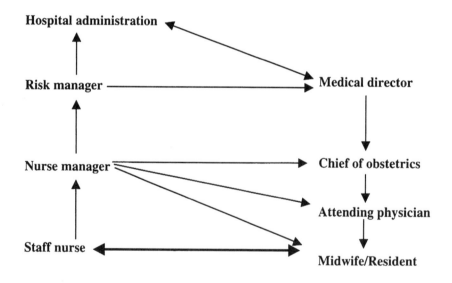

Figure 6-4. Example of problem resolution relying on chain of command.

Note: Some institutions have an ethics committee which might be included in some circumstances, time permitting.

Documentation

Documentation in fetal heart monitoring has the essential purposes of coordinating and communicating patient care and ensuring professional accountability. Whether auscultation or EFM is used, care providers are required to document their activities according to national professional standards, the Joint Commission on the Accreditation of Healthcare Organizations (JCAHO) or Canadian Council on Health Services Accreditation (CCHSA) guidelines, state or provincial regulations, and institutional protocols and procedures. Documentation also is used to demonstrate that the standard of care has been met.

Documentation of the FHR characteristics and the patterns requires the nurse to use appropriate descriptive terms of FHM whenever possible, record the status and changes of FHR characteristics and patterns, and describe the interventions used and responses (NAACOG, 1990; AWHONN, 1992). Documentation of FHM events follows many of the principles of charting: detailing what is heard, seen, felt, and smelled, as well as relaying clinical findings and demonstrating compliance with current standards of care (NAACOG, 1987a).

Principles of charting and documentation should be reviewed according to all relevant standards, related protocols, and nurse practice acts. All standard documentation principles apply to FHM documentation and should be used. When errors of charting were studied, five errors often appeared in charts that came to litigation:

- Incomplete initial history and physical

- Failure to observe and take appropriate action

- Failure to communicate changes in the condition of the patient

- Incomplete or inadequate documentation

- Failure to use or interpret fetal monitoring data appropriately.

(Chagnon & Easterwood, 1986)

Consideration of the following points when charting will help prevent the described errors, improve the quality of content, and decrease liability that is due to poor documentation (Grabenstein, 1987):

- All health care providers must be identifiable by their signature (first initial, full last name, and title).

- All entries are chronological and include a full date and time of entry. If an entry is made out of sequence, that entry should be labeled as a late entry and contain the date and time.

- A reviewer should be able to determine from the nursing notes the reason for hospitalization and/or intervention, the treatment provided, the results of the treatment, and the condition of the patients (mother and fetus).

- Factual documentation should include all direct observations and actions without omitting any significant facts.

191

- Documentation should be objective.

- Documentation should be legible.

- Documentation should be as specific as possible (e.g., STV and LTV, responses to position changes, vaginal exam findings).

- Documentation should include a description of the patient's ability to cope and apparent emotional response to labor and delivery.

- Documentation should include teaching and explanations given to patient and support people and their responses and apparent understanding.

Documentation Systems

Current systems used to document the patient's record include labor flow sheets, computerized programs, and charting by exception. These methods are cost-effective and avoid duplication of information. Clinical pathways also may be a useful tool for documentation of selected aspects of care (Simpson & Chez, 1996). Many formats and methods, from flow sheets to progress notes, from pen and paper charting to electronic/computer charting, are available to the nurse. Some hospitals continue to use narrative notes for documenting patient care and treatment. However, narrative notes alone lack specificity about maternal and fetal responses to labor and interventions employed by the nurse. It is easy to omit data, especially routine care if narrative notes are used exclusively. Labor flow sheets that are specific to the unit or institution provide better potential for thorough documentation. Flow sheets contribute to making documentation organized, understandable, and consistent. Labor flow sheets, which contain narrative notes as needed, are often effective and help to summarize maternal and fetal condition, plan of care, interventions, and response to care (Regan, 1987). Computerized systems, including bedside terminals, also may foster ease and efficiency in charting during the perinatal period. The method of charting by exception is dependent on individual institution policy for the way data are to be documented. For documentation to be useful, it must be easily read, understood, and retrievable.

When EFM is employed, an additional document, the tracing or laser disk, should be available for information and may be used for annotation. Words and symbols written on the tracing may be made by pen, keyboard, or scan, depending on the type of technology in use. Annotations are more accurate and useful when the time of entry is marked on the tracing by using the "mark" button. Indicating the exact time of entry may be helpful when the timing of the event may influence the FHR.

Clear documentation in the labor record that demonstrates that the standard of care is being met often may be accomplished without documenting in multiple sites. Charting of information in multiple locations is to be avoided whenever possible. The goal is to maximize time available for direct patient care and to minimize the likelihood of errors of transcription of information in multiple sites. Key elements for concise documentation include user-friendly systems that emphasize "hands-on" care as opposed to increased paper work. For example, some computer systems allow documentation of information in one location with automatic inclusion of the same information in other pertinent locations.

While documenting in multiple locations is to be avoided whenever possible, there may be specific situations where it is helpful to document directly on the fetal heart rate tracing. For example, it is appropriate in a situation that is rapidly unfolding to document directly on the tracing. A summary note may be entered on the labor record at a later time with the times of events within the body of the note. Some computer systems used for storage of tracings may not retain notes made on the tracings. It is important to know the capabilities and limitations of the particular documentation system in use to ensure that key information is retrievable from the maternal-fetal record.

Documentation should take place as events occur. Use of institution-specific forms without preprinted time intervals allows for more accurate documentation of events and their timing (Simpson & Chez, 1996).

Hospital policies for permanent storage of fetal heart tracings and medical record safekeeping vary according to specific hospital procedure and available technology. Technology for storage may be hard copy, microfilm techniques, or computer laser disk. Whatever the policy or technology, the "tracing is a legal part of the medical record including identifying information about the patient, as well as times and events related to the patient's ongoing care . . . " (AWHONN, 1992). The importance of the tracing in the documentation of appropriate patient care, and thus in the potential defense of hospital and involved caregivers, cannot be overemphasized.

Terminology

Documentation of fetal heart characteristics and patterns will be affected by the mode of monitoring employed (Figure 6-6), as well as by institutional forms, policies, and protocols. Documentation of auscultation uses specific terms designed to accurately and realistically describe the audible fetal heart rate, rhythm, and changes (Figure 6-5). Documentation of palpated uterine activity generally includes the terms mild, moderate, and strong. The words indentable and nonindentable are used to teach palpation of the fundus rather than for documentation. For example, a nonindentable fundal contraction is "strong." A sample flow sheet for documentation for charting auscultation and palpation is provided (Figure 6-7). Alternately, a sample of narrative for charting auscultation and palpation follows.

FHR 140's by auscultation with fetoscope, regular rhythm. Increase of FHR to 160 for 20 sec. during UC, returning to BL by end of UC. UCs every 3-4 min. X 50-60 sec., moderate, RT relaxed.

When using EFM, it is appropriate to use the descriptive names for FHR patterns including early, late, and variable decelerations (AWHONN, 1992). Variability may be documented according to the type of EFM in use (Figure 6-6). Complete, concise, and legible documentation cannot be overemphasized (Grabenstein, 1987). It is advisable to use standard abbreviations and for each institution to be in agreement on the accepted abbreviations to foster clear communication. Some

193

examples of commonly used abbreviations are provided (Table 6-1). Although samples are provided, abbreviations should be institution-specific and included in unit policy manuals and/or on the labor flow sheets.

Whatever the format and method employed for documentation, the content provides an adequate description of the fetal heart rate data so the reader can visualize or reasonably reproduce the pattern on paper. Use of some terms, such as asphyxia, hypoxia, and fetal distress, should be avoided in documentation. These terms are not precise or specific, and have little positive predictive value (ACOG, 1994, 1995).

Documentation of Fetal Heart Auscultation and Uterine Palpation

Fetal Heart Rate (FHR)

FH --- Numerical rate and rhythm (rhythm with fetoscope)

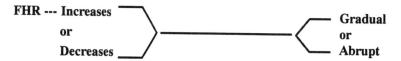

FHR --- Increases
or
Decreases
Gradual
or
Abrupt

Uterine Activity (UA)

UA --- Frequency and Duration

UA --- Intensity   **Mild**   **UA --- Tone Relaxed/Soft**
    Moderate   **Tense**
    Strong

Figure 6-5. Documentation of fetal heart auscultation and uterine palpation (NAACOG, 1990).

Documentation of Fetal Heart by Mode Employed

Auscultation	Ultrasound	Spiral Electrode
Rate	Rate	Rate
Rhythm	Rhythm	Rhythm
----	LTV	LTV
----	----	STV*
----	Periodic Patterns	Periodic Patterns
----	Nonperiodic Patterns	Nonperiodic Patterns
Increases/decreases		
• Abrupt		
• Gradual		

*   Although the technology of autocorrelation has improved the fetal heart tracing, more studies of autocorrelation validity and reliability are needed before documenting STV by ultrasound. This is especially critical when other reassuring features are absent from the tracing.

Documentation of Uterine Contraction by Mode Employed

Palpation	Tocodynamometer	Intrauterine Pressure Catheter (IUPC)
Frequency	Frequency	Frequency
Duration	Duration	Duration
Tonus	----	Tonus - actual
Intensity	----	Intensity - actual

Figure 6-6.   Documentation of fetal heart and uterine contraction by mode employed.

Frequency of Documentation

Frequency of documentation for women in latent labor is an institutional policy that may vary from 1 to 2 hours or per physician's or midwife's orders. High-risk antepartum patients not in labor will be assessed per hospital policy, which may be every 4 hours or according to specific physician's or midwife's orders.

ACOG states that the frequency of documentation of the FHR by auscultation for a low-risk intrapartum patient should be every 30 minutes during active phase of the first stage of labor and every 15 minutes during the second stage of labor. The high-risk intrapartum patient's fetus should be auscultated and documented every 15 minutes during the active phase of the first stage of labor and every 5 minutes during the second stage of labor (ACOG, 1995). In Canada, the recommended frequency of documentation is every 30 minutes during the latent phase, every 15 to 30 minutes in active phase, and every 5 minutes in the second stage with auscultation (SOGC, 1995). Documentation may occur at the same intervals or be summarized at longer intervals (AWHONN, 1992). Most institutions require the frequency for assessment of electronic fetal heart patterns to be the same or similar to the requirements for auscultation. Selected documentation examples based on EFM tracings are included (Figures 6-7 through 6-13).

DATE OF RECORD	2/3/96				
	TIME		12:00		
		:05			
CERVIX	Dilatation				
	Effacement				
	Station				
UTERINE ACTIVITY	Monitor Mode	Palp			
	Frequency	3 - 4			
	Duration	50 - 60			
	Intensity	Mod			
	Resting Tone	Soft			
FETAL	Monitor Mode	Ausc			
	FHR	140s/Reg			
	LTV				
	STV				
	Accelerations	to 160			
	Decelerations				
	STIM/pH				
	Maternal Position				
	O2/LPM/Mask				
	IV				
	NURSE INITIALS	NPX			

Figure 6-7. Sample of flow sheet charting of auscultation and palpation.

Examples of Abbreviations for Charting Fetal Monitoring

EFM	Electronic fetal monitor(ing)
FHR	Fetal heart rate
US	Ultrasound (external)
TOCO	Tocodynamometer (external)
SE	Spiral electrode (internal)
IUPC	Intrauterine pressure catheter (internal)
UC	Uterine contraction
BL	Baseline (refers to FHR, and sometimes baseline tonus)
bpm	Beats per minute
LTV +	Long-term variability average, within normal limits (WNL), 6-25 beats amplitude and 3-6 cycle changes/minute
LTV ↓	Long-term variability decreased, diminished, <0--5 bpm amplitude and <3 cycle changes/minute
LTV ↑	Long-term variability marked, saltatory, >25 beats amplitude and >6 cycle changes/minute
STV +	Short-term variability present; roughness of tracing line present
STV φ	Short-term variability absent; tracing line is smooth
Accel.	Acceleration of the FHR above the baseline rate
LD, Late decel	Late deceleration
ED, Early decel	Early deceleration
VD, Var decel	Variable deceleration
PD	Prolonged deceleration, lasting over 2 minutes
RT	Resting tone
UC,1+,2+,3+	Uterine contraction tone: Mild=M or 1+, Moderate Firm=MF or 2+, or Firm =F or 3+
MVU	Montevideo Units = total contraction intensity in mm HG minus the resting tone pressure of each contraction over 10 minutes
AFI	Amniotic fluid index
AST	Acoustic Stimulation Test
VAS	Vibracoustic Stimulation Test
AUSC	Auscultation
FM	Fetal movement
IUP	Intrauterine pressure
VE	Vaginal exam
REG	Regular
STIM	Scalp stimulation
NP	Nonperiodic
P	Periodic
UA	Uterine activity
avg	Average
dec	Decreased
inc	Increased
pos	Positive
neg	Negative

Table 6-1. Selected abbreviations for charting fetal monitoring. (Adapted from Schmidt, 1987; Tucker, 1996).

Note: There are other acceptable abbreviation choices for charting fetal monitoring. This table simply represents some of the commonly used abbreviations and is not intended to be all inclusive. Abbreviations should be institution-specific and included in the policy manuals and/or labor flow sheets.

198

Tracing and Documentation

DATE OF RECORD ___3/22/96___

		TIME	12:00			
			:15			
CERVIX	Dilatation					
CERVIX	Effacement					
CERVIX	Station					
UTERINE ACTIVITY	Monitor Mode		IUPC			
UTERINE ACTIVITY	Frequency		2 1/2 - 3			
UTERINE ACTIVITY	Duration		50 - 70			
UTERINE ACTIVITY	Intensity		65 - 70			
UTERINE ACTIVITY	Resting Tone		10			
FETAL	Monitor Mode		SE			
FETAL	FHR		140 - 155			
FETAL	LTV		+			
FETAL	STV		+			
FETAL	Accelerations		180			
FETAL	Decelerations		Var			
FETAL	STIM/pH					
	Maternal Position					
	O2/LPM/Mask					
	IV					
	NURSE INITIALS		smg			

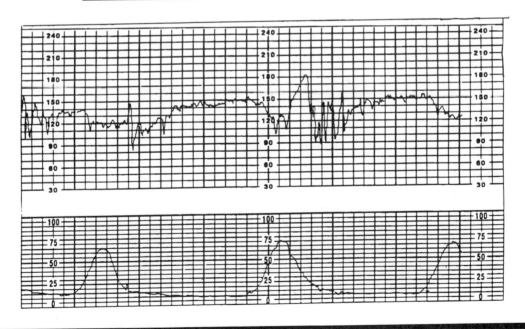

Figure 6-8. EFM documentation: SE and IUPC

DATE OF RECORD		1/1/97			
	TIME		2:00		
		:05			
CERVIX	Dilatation				
	Effacement				
	Station				
UTERINE ACTIVITY	Monitor Mode	TOCO			
	Frequency	2 - 2 1/2			
	Duration	70-90			
	Intensity	Palp/Mild			
	Resting Tone	Palp/Soft			
FETAL	Monitor Mode	US			
	FHR	140 - 150			
	LTV	+			
	STV	N/A			
	Accelerations	Ø			
	Decelerations	Var			
	STIM/pH				
	Maternal Position				
	O2/LPM/Mask				
	IV				
NURSE INITIALS		XJ			

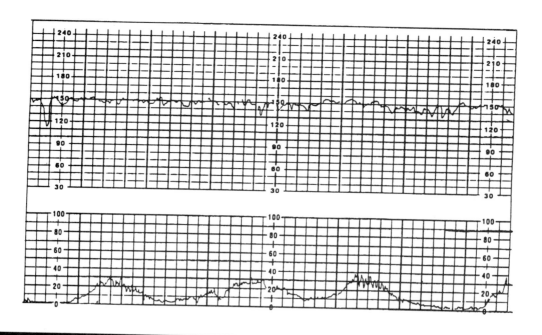

Figure 6-9. EFM documentation: US and toco

		TIME	2:00			
			:10			
CERVIX	Dilatation					
	Effacement					
	Station					
UTERINE ACTIVITY	Monitor Mode		**TOCO**			
	Frequency		1 1/2 - 2 1/2			
	Duration		70 - 130 - **Coupling**			
	Intensity		**Palp/Mod**			
	Resting Tone		**Palp/Soft**			
FETAL	Monitor Mode		**SE**			
	FHR		**95-100***			
	LTV		↓			
	STV		Ø			
	Accelerations		Ø			
	Decelerations					
	STIM/pH					
	Maternal Position					
	O2/LPM/Mask		**10L**			
	IV					
	NURSE INITIALS		SMD			

DATE OF RECORD 3/10/97

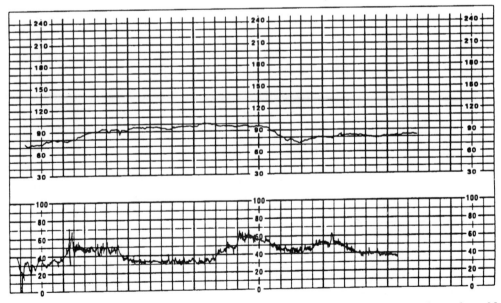

Narrative Note: 2:10 Prolonged bradycardia continues. Dr. here. Indwelling catheter placed. Surgical prep done. Monitor connections unplugged. Moved to OR for CS. N. Nurse, RN.

Figure 6-10. EFM documentation: SE and toco

DATE OF RECORD ___1/1/97___

		TIME	3:00			
			:15			
CERVIX	Dilatation		5 cms	Per OTM		
CERVIX	Effacement		100 %			
CERVIX	Station		0			
UTERINE ACTIVITY	Monitor Mode		IUPC			
UTERINE ACTIVITY	Frequency		2 1/2			
UTERINE ACTIVITY	Duration		60 - 90			
UTERINE ACTIVITY	Intensity		70 - 80			
UTERINE ACTIVITY	Resting Tone		15 - 20			
FETAL	Monitor Mode		SE			
FETAL	FHR		130 - 140			
FETAL	LTV		+			
FETAL	STV		+			
FETAL	Accelerations		160 - 165			
FETAL	Decelerations		Ø			
FETAL	STIM/pH		Ø			
	Maternal Position		RL			
	O2/LPM/Mask					
	IV					
	NURSE INITIALS		JRX			

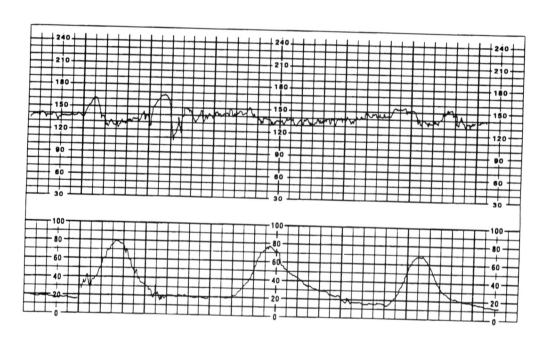

Figure 6-11. EFM documentation: SE and IUPC (NOTE: RL=Right lateral)

DATE OF RECORD		12/25/96			
	TIME		5:00		
		:05			
CERVIX	Dilatation				
	Effacement				
	Station				
UTERINE ACTIVITY	Monitor Mode	TOCO			
	Frequency	2 1/2 - 3			
	Duration	45 - 50			
	Intensity	Palp/Mild			
	Resting Tone	Palp/Soft			
FETAL	Monitor Mode	US			
	FHR	170 - 175			
	LTV	↓			
	STV	N/A			
	Accelerations	Ø			
	Decelerations	Ø			
	STIM/pH				
	Maternal Position				
	O2/LPM/Mask				
	IV				
	NURSE INITIALS	CRW			

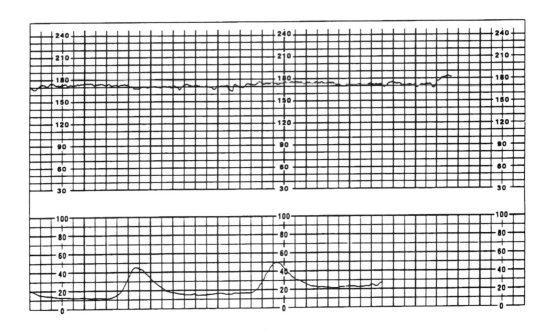

Figure 6-12. EFM documentation: US and toco

DATE OF RECORD 2/14/96					
TIME		10:00			
		:15			
CERVIX — Dilatation					
Effacement					
Station					
UTERINE ACTIVITY — Monitor Mode		IUPC			
Frequency		6 1/2 - 7			
Duration		70			
Intensity		35			
Resting Tone		10			
FETAL/BABY A — Monitor Mode		SE			
FHR		160 - 165			
LTV		↓			
STV		+			
Accelerations		175			
Decelerations		Ø			
STIM/pH					
FETAL/BABY B — Monitor Mode		US			
FHR		140 - 150			
LTV		+			
STV		N/A			
Accelerations		165 - 175			
Decelerations		Var			
STIM/pH					
Maternal Position					
O2/LPM/Mask					
IV					
NURSE INITIALS		JSW			

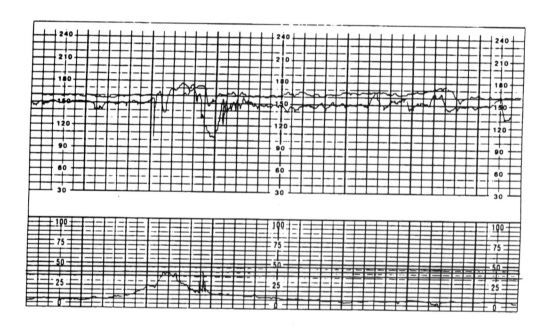

Figure 6-13. EFM documentation of twins

REFERENCES

ACOG. (1994). <u>Committee opinion: Fetal distress and birth asphyxia.</u> Washington, DC: Author.

ACOG. (1995) <u>Fetal heart rate patterns: Monitoring, interpretation, and management.</u> ACOG Technical Bulletin No. 207. Washington, DC: Author.

AWHONN. (1992). <u>Nursing responsibilities in implementing intrapartum fetal heart rate monitoring,</u> (Position Statement). Washington, DC: Author.

Chagnon, L., & Easterwood, B. (1986). Managing the risks of obstetrical nursing. <u>Maternal Child Nursing, 11,</u> 303-310.

Chez, B. F., Harvey, C. J., & Murray, M. L. (1990). <u>Critical concepts in fetal heart rate monitoring: Resources, guidelines, documentation.</u> Baltimore: Williams & Wilkins.

Enkin, M., Keirse, M., Renfrew, M., & Nelson, J. (1995). <u>A guide to effective care in pregnancy & childbirth</u> (2nd ed.). Oxford: Oxford University Press.

Grabenstein, J. (1987). Nursing documentation during the perinatal period. <u>Journal of Perinatal and Neonatal Nursing, 1</u>(2), 29-38.

Marquis, B. L., & Huston, C. J. (1992). <u>Leadership roles and management functions in nursing: Theory and application.</u> Philadelphia: J. B. Lippincott Company.

NAACOG. (1987a). Charting, documentation, and record-keeping. <u>Professional Liability Series.</u> Washington, DC: Author.

NAACOG. (1987b). Informed consent. <u>Professional Liability Series.</u> Washington, DC: Author.

NAACOG. (1987c). Medical orders and MD/RN communication. <u>Professional Liability Series.</u> Washington, DC: Author.

NAACOG. (1990). <u>Fetal heart rate auscultation,</u> OGN Nursing Practice Resource. Washington, DC: Author.

NAACOG. (1991). <u>Nursing practice competencies and educational guidelines: Antepartum fetal surveillance and intrapartum fetal heart monitoring</u> (2nd ed.). Washington, DC: Author.

Regan, M. T. (1987). Documentation for the defense. <u>Journal of Perinatal and Neonatal Nursing, 1</u>(2), 49-60.

Schmidt J. (1987). Documenting EFM events. <u>Perinatal Press, 10.</u>

Simpson, K. R., & Chez, B. F. (1996). Professional and legal issues. In K. R. Simpson & Creehan (Eds.), <u>Perinatal Nursing</u> (pp. 15-25). Philadelphia: Lippincott-Raven.

Society of Obstetricians and Gynaecologists of Canada (SOGC). (1995). SOGC Policy Statement: Fetal health surveillance in labour. Journal of SOGC, 17(9), 865-901.

Tucker, S. M. (1996). Fetal monitoring and assessment (3rd ed.). St. Louis: Mosby.

BIBLIOGRAPHY

(including resources on legal issues)

Afriat, C. I. (1983). The nurse's role in fetal heart rate monitoring. Perinatology Neonatology, 7(3), 29-32.

Albarado, R. S., McCall, V., & Thrane, J. M. (1990). Computerized nursing documentation. Nursing Management, 21(7), 64-65.

ACOG. (1990). Professional liability and its effects: Report of a 1990 survey of ACOG's membership. Washington, DC: Opinion Research Corporation.

ACOG. (1989). Intrapartum fetal heart rate monitoring, ACOG Technical Bulletin No. 132. Washington, DC: Author.

Blank, J. J. (1985). Electronic fetal monitoring: Nursing management defined. Journal of Obstetric, Gynecologic, and Neonatal Nursing, 14, 463-467.

Bolos, M. (1990). Rules of the game. In R. D. Eden & F. H. Boehm (Eds.), Assessment and care of the fetus (pp. 921-930). Norwalk, CT: Appleton & Lange.

Borten, M., & Freidman, E. (1990). Legal principles and practice in obstetrics and gynecology. Volume II. Chicago: Year Book Medical Publications.

Cetrulo, C. L., & Cetrulo, L. G. (1990). The medical chart. In R. D. Eden & F. H. Boehm (Eds.), Assessment and care of the fetus (pp. 961-964). Norwalk, CT: Appleton & Lange.

Cohn, S. D. (1987). Trends in perinatal nursing professional liability. Journal of Perinatal and Neonatal Nursing, 1(2), 19-27.

Cohn, S. D. (1990). Malpractice and liability in obstetrical nursing. Rockville, MD: Aspen Publishers, Inc.

Comstock, L. G., & Moff, T. (1991). Cost effective, time efficient charting. Nursing Management, 22(7), 44-48.

Creighton, H. (1986). Laws every nurse should know. Philadelphia: W. B. Saunders Company.

Divoli, M. K. (1987). The role of the perinatal and neonatal nurse in risk management. Journal of Perinatal and Neonatal Nursing, 1(2), 1-8.

Eganhouse, D. J. (1991). Electronic fetal monitoring education and quality assurance. Journal of Obstetric, Gynecologic, and Neonatal Nursing, 20, 16-22.

Ellin, M., Tafero, S. J., & Logan, R. J. (1990). Judge, jury, and you (Audiotape). Audio-Digest of Obstetrics and Gynecology, 37(20).

Fields, L. M. (1987). Electronic fetal monitoring: Practices and protocols for the intrapartum patient. Journal of Perinatal Neonatal Nursing, 1, 5-12.

Fields, L. M., & Boehm, F. H. (1989). Changing issues in fetal heart rate monitoring. Contemporary OB/GYN, 33(Suppl.), 145.

Fiesta, J. (1991). If it wasn't charted, it wasn't done. Nursing Management, 22(8), 17.

Flanigan, L. (1990). Survival skills in the workplace: What every nurse should know. Kansas City, MO: American Nurses' Association.

Gilstrap, L. C., & Depp, R. (1990). Medicolegal alert (Audiotape). Audio Digest of Obstetrics and Gynecology, 37(5).

Halawelka, M. (1991). This doctor owed $15 million in malpractice damages. Medical Economics, 68(1), 96-112.

Hardy, J. C., & Douglas, M. (1990). High-tech nurse stations on nursing units. Nursing Management, 21, 7.

Hickson, G. B., Clayton, E. W., Githens, P. B., & Sloan, F. A. (1992). Factors that prompted families to file medical malpractice claims following perinatal injuries. Journal of the American Medical Association, 267, 1359-1363.

Machol, L. (1989). Facsimile telecopiers keep improving. Contemporary OB/GYN, 34(Suppl.), 53.

Murray, M. (1988). Antepartal and intrapartal fetal monitoring. Washington, DC: NAACOG.

NAACOG. (1990). Fetal heart rate auscultation, OGN Nursing Practice Resource. Washington, DC: Author.

Perlow, J. H., & Garite, T. J. (1991). Update on electronic fetal monitoring systems. Contemporary OB/GYN, 36(Suppl.), 44.

Phelan, J. P., Freeman, R. K., Gargaro, W. J., & O'Keye, D. (1991). Confronting medical liability. Contemporary OB/GYN, 36, 70-81.

Robbins, D. (1987). Incident report analysis: The experience of one large labor and delivery unit. Journal of Perinatal and Neonatal Nursing, 1, 9-18.

Ryan, M. A. (1989). Legal aspects of obstetrical nursing: Implications of the obstetrical record (Teleconference). Fairfield, CT: Quality Assurance Associates.

Sarno, A. P., Phelan, J. P., & Ohm, M. O. (1990). Relationship of early intrapartum fetal heart rate patterns to subsequent patterns and fetal outcome. American Journal of Obstetrics and Gynecology. 35, 239.

Schifrin, B. S. (1990). The patient as plaintiff. In R. D. Eden & F. H. Boehm (Eds.), <u>Assessment and care of the fetus</u> (pp. 971-976). Norwalk, CT: Appleton & Lange.

Sims, M. E. (1991). Dating the brain injury. <u>Contemporary OB/GYN</u>, <u>36</u>, 53-57.

Sullivan, G. H. (1989). <u>Legal aspects of obstetrical nursing: What every obstetrical nurse should know about malpractice liability</u> (Teleconference). Fairfield, CT: Quality Assurance Associates.

Tammello, A. D. (1991). Failure to use fetal monitor and timely call physician. Case in point: Garcia v. Providence Medical Center (806 P. 2d 766-WA [1991]). <u>Regan Report Nursing Law, 31</u>.

Tammello, A. D. (1987). Nurses' notes: Worth weight in gold. <u>Regan Report Nursing Law, 27</u>.

Ward, C. J. (1991). Analysis of 500 obstetric and gynecologic malpractice claims: Causes and prevention. <u>American Journal of Obstetrics and Gynecology, 165</u>, 139-145.

CHAPTER 7: SUMMARY

This manual has provided a historical and contemporary overview of fetal heart monitoring practice, education, and the AWHONN FHMPP workshop. Chapters have provided information on fetal and maternal physiology, assessment techniques, instrumentation for technological monitoring, interpretation of fetal heart monitoring data, independent and collaborative intervention, and communication methods. The nursing process model has been the framework for the content. Content has emphasized key principles of fetal heart monitoring necessary for practice including

- Significance of fetal and maternal physiology

- Significance of fetal and maternal history

- Importance of the critical decision-making process for selecting and verifying fetal assessment techniques

- Interpretation of patterns and their implications for fetal well-being

- Correlation of clinical interventions and related physiology

- Evaluation of fetal-maternal response to intervention

- Communication, including written, verbal, and conflict resolution

- Accountability and role of the professional nurse in fetal monitoring.

A systematic approach to cognitive analysis of FHR data has been presented. The skill of systematic analysis initially is a process of conscious individual steps. With experience, the skill becomes a process of integration with increasingly automatic, simultaneous steps.

To complete the workshop, the problem-based didactic and skill sessions will enable the participant to demonstrate integration of cognitive knowledge and psychomotor skills.

CHAPTER 8: GLOSSARY OF KEY TERMS

Acceleration -- A transitory increase in the fetal heart rate from the baseline rate. Associated with sympathetic nervous stimulation.

Acidemia -- An abnormal excess of hydrogen ion concentration in the blood that is due to increased acid build up or increased loss of base.

Acidosis -- An abnormal excess hydrogen ion concentration in tissues that is due to increased acid buildup or increased loss of base.

Alkalosis -- An increase in pH value (decreased hydrogen ion concentration) above normal.

Alpha-fetoprotein test (AFP test) -- A test indicating level of AFP in maternal serum or amniotic fluid. AFP is a glycoprotein in fetal serum. Elevated levels in maternal serum may be associated with increased risk of neural tube defects; low levels may be associated with risk of Down's Syndrome or other chromosomal abnormalities. Fetal levels peak at 15 weeks; maternal levels peak at 30 weeks. Results may be affected by gestational age, race, maternal weight, multiple gestation, and insulin-dependent diabetes.

Amnioinfusion -- Installation of fluid into the uterus through an intrauterine catheter. Used to increase amniotic fluid volume in situations of oligohydramnios or umbilical cord compression with associated variable decelerations. Also used to dilute amniotic fluid in situations of meconium stained amniotic fluid.

Amniotic fluid index (AFI) -- The amount of amniotic fluid measured by ultrasonography in centimeters of visible fluid.

Amplitude -- The distance between high and low points of the FHR tracing oscillations. Used in reference to long term variability range in beats per minute.

Apt test -- Distinguishes fetal and maternal red blood cells in a maternal or neonatal specimen (e.g., vaginal blood flow, meconium, or gastric aspirate). A qualitative test.

Arrhythmia -- Irregular, abnormal heart action or absence of rhythm. Associated with alteration in transmission of cardiac impulses. Sometimes used interchangeably with dysrhythmia.

Artifact -- Irregular variation or absence of FHR on the fetal monitor tracing that is due to mechanical limitations or electrical interference of the monitoring system.

Asphyxia -- Decrease in oxygen in body tissue (hypoxia), increase in CO_2 level (hypercapnia), and decrease in pH (metabolic and/or respiratory acidosis) with buildup of lactic acid in the tissue.

Atrial flutter -- Tachycardiac FHR (often from 300 to 460 beats per minute) which often exhibits a 2:1 atrioventricular block by echocardiography and half-counting by EFM.

Atrial fibrillation -- Tachycardiac atrial FHR (often from 300-460 beats per minute) rarely identified in the fetus.

Auscultation -- An auditory assessment procedure or process of listening for sounds within the body, such as fetal heart sounds. Fetal heart sounds are auscultated to determine rate and rhythm. True auscultation is performed with a fetoscope, or stethoscope (e.g. Pinard), but this term frequently is used to include the use of a hand-held Doppler ultrasound device to detect FHR.

Autocorrelation -- Microprocessor comparison of consecutive points of waveforms generated by the electronic fetal monitor. Comparison is based on ultrasound waves reflected from the moving fetal heart valves. Mechanism in second-generation fetal monitors.

Baroreceptor -- Pressure-sensitive stretch receptor in carotid sinus and aortic arch that responds to blood pressure changes by altering the FHR via the sympathetic (increase in rate) and parasympathetic (decrease in rate) nervous system.

Base deficit -- Measures the amount of base buffer reserves below normal levels. A large positive base deficit (e.g., 10 mEq/liter) indicates that base buffers have been used to buffer acids, that sufficient base reserves are not present, and that metabolic acidosis is present.

Base excess -- Measures the amount of base buffers reserves above normal levels. A large negative base excess (e.g., -10 mEq/liter) indicates that base buffers have been used to buffer acids, that sufficient base reserves are not present, and that metabolic acidosis is present.

Baseline fetal heart rate -- Average FHR over 10 minutes, between uterine contractions, decelerations, or accelerations.

Bishop Score -- A method for determining cervical readiness for induction of labor by scoring 5 components: cervical dilation, effacement, consistency, position, and station of the presenting part. Higher score is associated with successful induction of labor. Score also has been used as an assessment in preterm labor suppression.

Bradyarrhythmia -- An irregular heart rate rhythm usually occurring when FHR is below 90 beats per minute (e.g., sinus bradycardia or heart block). Visualized by fetal echocardiography or ECG.

Bradycardia -- Baseline FHR below 110 beats per minute for longer than 10 minutes. Slow heart action.

Certification -- The process by which an organization documents an individual's knowledge in a nursing specialty.

Chemoreceptor -- Sensory nerve endings or organs stimulated by a chemical response. Sensitive to change in oxygen, carbon dioxide, and pH levels in the blood.

Combined deceleration patterns -- Visual patterns resulting when more than one physiologic mechanism occurs that cause a combination of "single" deceleration patterns in regard to shape and timing. Contains characteristics of both of the single patterns in regard to shape and timing.

Compensatory response to hypoxemia -- Describes the ability of the fetus to adjust to low blood oxygen levels by drawing from fetal reserves. The presence of STV implies fetal reserves.

Competence validation -- Verification of knowledge and skills according to predetermined criteria.

Conflict resolution -- Process of resolving professional disagreements within the mechanisms of institutional policies, procedures, and protocols. Process may involve implementing the chain of command.

Deceleration -- A transitory decrease in the FHR from the baseline rate.

Doppler -- Generally refers to a hand-held instrument that emits ultrasound waves. It converts the waves reflected from the moving fetal heart into a fetal heart rate.

Dysrhythmia -- A fetal heart rhythm that is associated with a disordered impulse formation, impulse conduction, or a combination of both.

Early deceleration -- A transitory decrease in the FHR from the baseline rate caused by compression of the fetal vertex during contractions and resultant vagal stimulation. Characterized by synchronous onset and offset with uterine contractions. Mirrors the contraction. Uniform in shape.

Electronic fetal monitoring -- An auditory and visual assessment of the FHR with data generated by fetal monitor technology. Generated data includes a digital or graphic display and a permanent record on paper or laser disk.

Extrinsic influences -- Factors outside the fetus that may affect the FHR characteristics (e.g., maternal, placental, or umbilical cord factors).

Favorable physiologic response -- A FHR response associated with a positive prognosis for fetal outcome; associated with a fetus that is able to respond appropriately to the environment and maintain fetal reserves.

Fetal reserve -- Additional amount of oxygen available to the fetus beyond the amount normally required by the fetus for metabolism.

Fetoscope -- Stethoscope adapted for auscultation of the FHR (also known as DeLee fetoscope).

First-generation monitor -- An electronic fetal monitor that uses a refractory window and peak-to-peak comparison of fetal heart waveforms generated by an external ultrasound transducer. Rate is calculated by averaging peaks.

Funic souffle (bruit) -- A soft "blowing" sound heard by auscultation over the umbilical cord. Synchronous with the FHR.

Heart block -- A condition in which the electrical impulses in the heart are not conducted normally from the atrium to the ventricles via the sinoatrial node, atrioventricular node, bundle of HIS, and Purkinje fibers. Results in bradycardia. May be intermittent.

Hydrostatic pressure -- The pressure exerted by a fluid in a closed system, such as pressure created by amniotic fluid in the uterus. An intrauterine pressure catheter (IUPC) measures hydrostatic pressure in the uterus during and between uterine contractions.

Hypoxemia -- Low levels of oxygen in the blood.

Hypoxia -- Low levels of oxygen available in the tissue, inadequate to meet metabolic needs of the tissue.

Impending decompensation -- The loss of the ability of the fetus to respond physiologically to the feto-maternal environment; may include a loss of fetal reserves and inability to maintain the heart rate.

Intermittent auscultation -- Listening to the FHR at periodic intervals either by fetoscope or handheld Doppler.

Intrauterine pressure catheter (IUPC) -- A catheter used to directly measure intrauterine pressure during and between uterine contractions. The catheter may be fluid filled or sensor tipped.

Intrinsic factors -- Internal fetal regulatory mechanisms that control the heart rate, including sympathetic, parasympathetic, and central nervous systems, baroreceptor, chemoreceptor, and hormonal responses.

Kleihauer-Betke test -- A blood analysis to detect the presence and relative amount of fetal hemoglobin in the maternal blood specimen. When blood specimen is stained on a slide, cells characterized with fetal hemoglobin can be viewed and counted to determine the ratio of fetal blood cells to maternal blood cells. Quantitative test.

Late deceleration -- A repetitive decrease in the FHR from the baseline rate caused by uteroplacental insufficiency. Deceleration is late in onset and in recovery in relationship to the uterine contraction and is uniform in shape. The decrease may be small or subtle, but still be significant.

Leopold's maneuvers -- A systematic method of abdominal palpation to assess the fetus and uterus. Maneuvers include four steps.

Long-term variability (LTV) -- Oscillatory changes in the FHR baseline. Most frequently described in terms of amplitude within the baseline range, but also includes frequency of oscillations (cycles) over 1 minute.

Medulla oblongata -- The lower portion of the brain stem; the relay center for the parasympathetic and sympathetic nervous system.

Metabolic acidosis -- Decrease in blood pH associated with an increase in hydrogen ions, decrease in PO_2, and increase in base deficit (base excess). The PCO_2 may be normal.

Metabolic alkalosis -- Increase in blood pH associated with a decrease in hydrogen ions and a decrease in PCO_2.

Mixed acidosis -- Combination of metabolic and respiratory acidosis, associated with a decrease in pH, decrease in PO_2, an increase in PCO_2 levels, and an increase in base deficit.

Montevideo units -- Total pressure in mm Hg for all uterine contractions within a 10-minute time frame. The baseline resting tone is subtracted from the peak uterine pressure for each contraction to determine the mm Hg.

Nadir -- The lowest FHR value in a deceleration or depth of a deceleration. With electronic monitoring, it is visually the lowest point in the deceleration curve.

Nonhypoxemic reflex response -- Refers to a FHR response to an event not associated with decreased PO_2. Fetus quickly responds to change caused by an event (e.g., baroreceptor and vagal response affecting fetal blood pressure because of brief compression of the umbilical cord).

Nonperiodic pattern -- Accelerations or decelerations of the FHR in response to isolated versus repetitive uterine contractions (e.g., deceleration or acceleration in response to vaginal exam, fetal movement, tetanic contraction, cord compression, or maternal vomiting).

Nonreassuring fetal heart rate pattern -- Pattern that reflects a presumed unfavorable physiologic fetal response to the feto-maternal environment. A descriptive term.

Overshoot -- Exaggerated compensatory increase in the FHR after a variable deceleration. Usually at least 20 bpm increase for a duration greater than 20 seconds. Nonreassuring when repetitive and without baseline variability.

Para (P) -- Number of pregnancies that have resulted in viable offspring. The TPAL method of describing parity refers to the number of term births (T), preterm births (P), abortions (A), and living children (L) (e.g., gravida 3, para 1102).

Parasympathetic nervous system -- Part of autonomic nervous system. Includes vagal nerves which decrease heart rate when stimulated.

Periodic pattern -- Accelerations or decelerations of the FHR that occur in direct association with uterine contractions.

Periodic accelerations -- Transitory increases in the FHR that occur repetitively and are associated with uterine contractions. May be attributed to fetal movement, mild partial umbilical cord compression, or sympathetic stimulation from fundal pressure on the fetal head in a breech presentation.

Piezoelectric effect -- The crystals in the ultrasound transducer generate sound waves that are reflected back from moving structures. A shift in frequency of the waveforms reflected will identify the FHR.

Postterm pregnancy -- Pregnancy lasting beyond 42 completed weeks of gestation.

Premature ventricular contraction (PVC) -- Premature depolarization in the heart with resultant irregularity in the heart rate and rhythm.

Prolonged deceleration -- Decrease in the fetal heart rate from the baseline for longer than 2 minutes but usually less than 10 minutes. Associated with stimuli, such as cord compression, uterine hypertonus, and response to medications.

Pseudosinusoidal pattern -- A "sawtooth" undulating FHR pattern associated with periods of normal variability (STV and LTV) and accelerations. Less smooth, less constant than sinusoidal pattern and thought to be benign.

Reactivity -- Presence of FHR accelerations meeting the criteria of 15 beats per minute increase over 15 seconds occurring at least twice in 20 minutes. Usually associated with normal variability.

Reassuring pattern -- Pattern that reflects a presumed favorable physiologic response to the feto-maternal environment. A descriptive term.

Refractory window -- An inhibitory period in which the electronic ultrasound transducer does not attempt to count the incoming signal. Mechanism in first-generation fetal monitors.

Reserves -- Oxygen available to the fetus for metabolism. The degree of hypoxemia the fetus can tolerate before true tissue hypoxia and acidosis occur.

Respiratory acidosis -- A decrease in pH associated with an increase in carbonic acid and increase in CO_2, while base deficit may be within normal range. If pulmonary or placental exchange is increased, the amount of CO_2 in the extracellular tissue may decrease.

Respiratory alkalosis -- An increase in pH associated with a decrease in hydrogen ions and a decrease in PCO_2 (often associated with hyperventilation).

Rhythm -- Regularity or irregularity of the baseline FHR.

Saltatory -- LTV that is greater than 25 bpm; also defined as marked LTV.

Second generation monitor -- An electronic ultrasound fetal monitor that uses multiple comparison points in the waveforms generated by the external ultrasound transducer. Rate calculated by autocorrelation.

Short-term variability (STV) -- Changes in the FHR from one beat to the next. Measures the R to R intervals in the fetal cardiac cycle (QRS). Presence reflects fetal reserves. Measured only by direct spiral electrode.

Shoulders -- Pre- and post-accelerations present with variable decelerations. Generally of short duration (20 seconds) and 5 to 15 bpm above the baseline. Not associated with poor outcome.

Sinusoidal pattern -- A persistent sine wave or recurrent undulating FHR pattern that is smooth (absent short-term variability), uniform, usually within the normal heart rate range, and without periods of normal FHR reactivity.

Solid sensor-tipped IUPC -- An intrauterine pressure catheter that has a microprocessor transducer at the catheter tip which measures the intrauterine pressure directly.

Spiral electrode -- An internal monitoring device applied directly to the fetal presenting part which receives signals from the electrocardiac impulses of the fetal heart. Used to directly determine FHR and STV based on changes in the R to R intervals in successive QRS complexes.

Strain gauge -- A pressure transducer that electronically converts uterine pressure changes exerted on a diaphragm into mm Hg. Component of closed pressure system using a fluid-filled intrauterine catheter.

Supraventricular tachycardia -- A rapid FHR (180-320 beats per minute) associated with fixed R to R intervals. Atrial in origin.

Sympathetic nervous system -- A part of the autonomic nervous system. Stimulation results in FHR increase.

Tachycardia -- Baseline FHR above 160 beats per minute for longer than 10 minutes.

Tachysystole -- Abnormally frequent uterine contractions.

Tocodynamometer (tocotransducer) -- An external monitor that detects changes in uterine shape through the abdomen. Provides information about relative frequency, duration, and shape of contractions.

Tonus -- Intensity of uterine tone or intrauterine pressure between uterine contractions.

Ultrasound transducer -- An external monitor that detects movement of the fetal heart valves opening and closing through transmission of a sound wave and Doppler shift. Monitor processor converts reflected sound waves into a FHR.

Undulating pattern -- A FHR pattern that has a characteristic repetitive sine wave shape. Includes sinusoidal and pseudosinusoidal patterns.

Unfavorable physiologic response -- A FHR response associated with a fetus that is unable to respond appropriately to the feto-maternal environment and is demonstrating a loss of fetal-reserves.

Uterine bruit -- The sound heard when listening to the blood flow in the maternal uterine vessels (also known as uterine souffle). Synchronous with maternal pulse.

Vaginal manipulation -- A vaginal exam performed to elevate fetal presenting part off the umbilical cord (e.g., in the presence of a prolapsed cord).

Variable deceleration -- An abrupt decrease in the FHR from the baseline rate associated with compression of the umbilical cord. Deceleration is irregular in shape, timing, and depth. May be associated with contractions (periodic) or not associated with contractions (nonperiodic).

Variability (baseline variability) -- Changes in the baseline FHR due to sympathetic and parasympathetic innervation. Generally used to describe beat-to-beat changes (STV) and oscillatory changes (LTV). Monitoring method determines which type of variability can be reliably described.

Ms Jackson - induction for postdates.

• Postdates.

P2

Started IV

Res. did bbgd mec fd.
nyprin (? tone)
deep variables c̄ contr
23 - 4 min   50-70 IUPS

• HR 140 reactyaverage v- (any decs?)

• Contr ↓ 50s

• how long? 20 min

bad bolus? mcus

bolus 800cc

? STV → didn't say
whether spontaneous or
nor

→

CHAPTER 9: SKILL STATIONS

Auscultation in Fetal Heart Monitoring

Objectives:

1. Determine accurate FHR and rhythm.

2. Indicate presence or absence of general increases or decreases from the FHR baseline.

3. Select appropriate nursing interventions based on auscultated FHR and rhythm.

Introductory Principles:

1. Use of auscultation requires the ability to integrate underlying physiology, maternal and fetal historical data, and physical assessment data with data gathered by auscultation.

2. Auscultation requires the development of auditory skills to establish baseline rates and identify changes in rate and rhythm.

3. Use of auscultation presumes knowledge and understanding of the indications, benefits, and limitations of this method of fetal assessment.

4. Auscultation provides another assessment perspective; data for interpretation of rate, rhythm, general increases or decreases in the FHR; and data for appropriate and timely interventions.

5. Use of auscultation presumes a nurse to fetus ratio of 1:1 to be considered as effective as the use of EFM during active labor.

Steps in Skill Performance:

This skill station focuses on the actual technique of auscultation to determine the FHR, rhythm, and abrupt increases or decreases in the rate. This information will be used to determine appropriate nursing interventions, including physiologic-based interventions and selection of alternate monitoring methods as appropriate.

1. Verbalize locating the site for auscultation over the fetal back.

2. Verbalize verification of the FHR by checking maternal pulse.

3. Count the FHR between uterine contractions for at least 30 to 60 seconds to identify a baseline rate.

4. Count the FHR during a contraction and for a minimum of 30 seconds after the contraction to assess changes in baseline rate.

5. If distinct changes in the rate are noted, count the FHR for longer periods as needed.

6. Record the rate, rhythm, and general increases or decreases in the FHR.

7.   Indicate appropriate interventions based on results, including physiologic-based actions or changes in monitoring methods if indicated.

Suggestions for Practicing Auscultation:

1.   Bring a watch to the workshop for the auscultation skill station.

2.   Counting the FHR for multiple brief intervals may provide a clearer "picture" of the FHR baseline. For example, count for 6 seconds and multiply by 10 for consecutive intervals. These numbers can be written on paper over time to create a visual image of the changes in the FHR (Table 9-1). A portion of fetal monitor paper also may be used. Counting for longer intervals results in averaging of the FHR over a longer period of time and may not reflect the changes occurring in the FHR.

3.   If an increase or decrease from the baseline is audible, begin counting again to distinguish the change from baseline.

4.   When the beginning of the contraction or end of a contraction is announced, begin counting again to detect rate changes if present.

5.   Remember that interventions based on your findings may include continuing current interventions (e.g., provide patient support; continue auscultation) or altering interventions (e.g., change maternal position; re-auscultate; change to ultrasound monitor to verify changes in FHR).

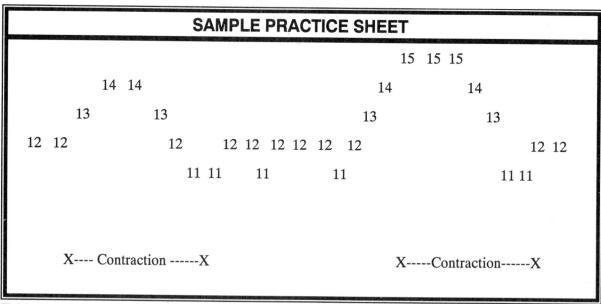

Table 9-1. Practice sheet for auscultating fetal heart rates (Read these steps before listening to the tapes)

Critical Errors in Testing:

1.   Failure to assess and document the FHR and rhythm for two patterns.

2.   Failure to document appropriate nursing interventions for the same two patterns.

Evaluation:

SKILL EVALUATION: **Auscultation in Fetal Heart Monitoring**

	Pass	**Fail**	**Date**
1. Assesses and documents FHR and rhythm for two fetuses.	___	___	___
2. Documents appropriate nursing interventions for the two FHR patterns auscultated.	___	___	___

Special thanks is extended to Marilyn R. Lapidus, RNC, BSN, Director, Clinical and Scientific Affairs, at Corometrics for her help in developing materials used in this skill station.

Abdominal Palpation in Fetal Heart Monitoring

Objectives:

In this skill station, the participant will

1. Explain Leopold's maneuvers and state patient comfort measures prior to the procedure.

2. Perform the four steps of Leopold's maneuvers.

3. Demonstrate accurate site for FHR auscultation based on assessment using Leopold's maneuvers.

Introductory Principles:

1. Evaluation of uterine tone, irritability, tenderness, consistency, and presence or absence of contractions can be obtained when performing palpation.

2. Fetal weight and fetal movement can be assessed during an abdominal examination.

3. The baby's lie (longitudinal, transverse, oblique), presentation (cephalic, breech, shoulder), and position (anterior, posterior, transverse, right, left) can be evaluated with Leopold's maneuvers and may be confirmed with a vaginal exam.

4. Correct placement of the instrument used for auscultating a FHR can be determined by completing Leopold's maneuvers.

5. Performing Leopold's maneuvers expedites location of FHR.

Steps in Skill Performance:

This skill station focuses on the skill in performing Leopold's maneuvers to determine the site for FHR auscultation. Patient education about the procedure and comfort measures also is included.

1. Steps in Skill Performance:

    (1) Patient comfort

        (a) Wash hands, warm them.
        (b) Instruct woman to empty bladder.
        (c) Expose abdomen from symphysis pubis to xiphoid process.
        (d) Drape woman appropriately.
        (e) Position woman with pillow under her head, knees flexed, and arms at her side.
        (f) Place small wedge under patient's right hip.
        (g) Explain the steps of the Leopold's maneuvers you will be performing.

(h) Place hands on woman's abdomen during your explanation so if her abdominal muscle becomes tense with your touch, it will have time to relax prior to your performing the maneuvers.

(2) Preparation for Leopold's maneuvers

    (a) Inspect abdomen for bulges (small parts), fetal movement, long axis of the baby.

    (b) Use flat, palmar surface of hands, with fingers together for a gentle but firm exam.

    (c) Stand at woman's right or left side, depending on your dominant side.

(3) Performing Leopold's maneuvers

    (a) Beginning with the first maneuver, face woman, with hands at top and side of the fundus. Be attentive to the size, shape, and consistency of what is in the fundus (note where longitudinal axis of baby is located).

    (b) For second maneuver, remain standing at the woman's side, facing her, with hands placed on either side at the middle of the abdomen. One hand will push the contents of the abdomen toward the other hand, to stabilize the baby for palpation. The hand that is doing the palpating begins at the middle of the abdomen near the fundus and moves posterior toward the woman's back. Repeat this process, progressing downward to the symphysis pubis. Determine which part of the baby lies on the side of the abdomen. If firm, smooth, and consistent, it is likely to be the back. If smaller, protruding, and irregular, it is likely to be the small parts. Note the location of the small parts and the back. Reverse the hands and repeat the maneuver.

    (c) With the third maneuver, remain facing the woman. With the middle finger and thumb grasp the part of the baby situated over the pelvic brim. With firm, gentle pressure determine if the head is the presenting part. This will confirm what you have felt in the first two maneuvers. If the presenting part moves, it is not engaged in the pelvis. If the presenting part is fixed and difficult to move, it is likely to be engaged. The third maneuver also is known as Pallach's maneuver/grip.

    (d) For the fourth maneuver, turn and face the woman's feet. Place your hands on the sides of her uterus, below the umbilicus, pointing toward the symphysis pubis. Press deeply, with fingertips toward the pelvic inlet, and feel for the cephalic prominence pubis. If the cephalic prominence is felt on the same side as the baby's back, it will be the occiput and the head will be slightly extended. If the cephalic prominence is felt on the same side as the small parts, it is likely to be the sinciput and the baby will be in a vertex or well-tucked position. If the cephalic prominence is felt equally on each side, it's the baby's head that will probably be in a military position, which is common when the baby is posterior. Finally, move the hands down toward the pelvic brim. If the hands come together around the presenting part, it indicates that the presenting part is floating. If the hands stay apart, the presenting part is either dipping or engaged in the pelvis.

(4) Share the information with the woman and ask if she would like to feel her baby through palpation, if appropriate.

(5) Locate and verify the FHR, which generally can be heard over the curved part of the baby closest to the anterior wall of the uterus.

(6) Document the findings of Leopold's maneuvers, the FHR and rhythm, and appropriate nursing interventions.

Definitions: The baby's	lie	position of long axis of fetus (longitudinal, transverse, oblique)
	presentation	that part of the fetus that lies over the pelvis (cephalic, breech, shoulder)
	position	relationship to maternal pelvis (anterior, posterior, transverse, right, left)
	attitude	relationship of fetal parts to each other (flexion, extension) can be evaluated with Leopold maneuvers and confirmed with the vaginal exam

Table 9-2. Leopold's maneuvers: Selected fetal assessments

Critical Errors in Testing:

1. Failure to explain the Leopold's maneuvers and state patient comfort measures prior to the procedure.

2. Failure to perform one of the four steps of the Leopold's maneuvers.

3. Failure to indicate optimal area for auscultation.

Evaluation:

SKILL EVALUATION: **Palpation in Fetal Heart Monitoring**

	Pass	Fail	Date
1. Explains Leopold's maneuvers and states patient comfort measures prior to procedure.	_____	_____	_____
2. Performs the four steps of the Leopold's maneuvers. (Assess part of fetus in the upper uterus, assess location of the fetal back, identify presenting part, and determine the descent of the presenting part.)	_____	_____	_____
3. Indicates optimal area for auscultation.	_____	_____	_____

Special thanks is extended to Childbirth Graphics, the staff at Fairview-Riverside Medical Center, Minneapolis, MN, and Melissa D. Avery, CNM, MSN, for their help in developing materials used in this skill station.

Instrumentation: Fetal Spiral Electrode and Intrauterine Pressure Catheter Placement

Objectives:

In this skill station, the participant will

1. Simulate correct placement of spiral electrode (SE).

2. Demonstrate safety principles related to placement of SE and intrauterine pressure catheter (IUPC).

3. Demonstrate correct sequence of steps related to placement and functioning of IUPC.

Introductory Principles:

1. Placement of the spiral electrode and intrauterine pressure catheter requires not only skills and techniques of vaginal examination and EFM but also knowledge of indications, risks, limitations, and contraindications.

2. These invasive procedures presume knowledge and understanding of

    *   maternal and fetal anatomy via vaginal palpation route.
    *   intrapartum changes.
    *   indications for direct measure of fetal heart dynamics or uterine dynamics.
    *   signs and symptoms of contraindications for direct, invasive monitoring.
    *   risks of employing direct monitoring modes, especially due to improper technique (e.g., hemorrhage, abruption, uterine perforation, and maternal and fetal infections).

3. The benefits of acquiring the actual electronic fetal cardiac data and uterine pressures provide another assessment perspective, data for interpretation, and data for appropriate, timely interventions.

Steps in Skill Performance:

This skill station focuses on the actual technique of placement and acknowledges the total process from approaching the patient to obtaining accurate data.

1. Spiral Electrode Placement

    The electrode usually is attached to the fetal scalp or buttock for direct measurement of the FHR by electrical activity. The spiral attaches approximately 2 mm into the presenting fetal part. The fetal lead detects the FHR electrical activity. The maternal reference electrode detects the maternal heart rate via her vaginal secretions or via placement of an external reference electrode. The external reference, when available, may be helpful when the signal is inadequate.

Procedure:

(1)   Explain procedure to mother prior to application.

(2)   Open electrode package and don gloves.

(3)   Remove wires from between drive tube and guide tube.

(4)   Pull electrode one inch back into guide tube so it does not extend beyond the end of guide.

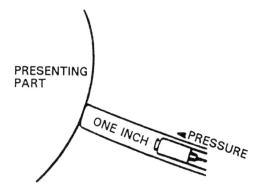

(5)   Perform vaginal exam to assess presenting part. Feel for firm bone and avoid face, fontanel, genitalia (see pictures attached); maintain fingers on target areas.

(6)   Place guide tube between two examining fingers and firmly place against fetal head at a right angle.

(7)   Advance drive tube until it touches the presenting part.

(8)   Maintain pressure against presenting part and turn clockwise (about 1 ½ times) until resistance is met.

(9)   Release lock device and slide guides of electrode.

(10)   Check placement of electrode before withdrawing examining fingers.

(11)   Attach monitor to cable device.

(12)   Verbalize that cable is plugged into monitor.

(13)   Verbalize documentation on tracing and medical record.

(14)   Verbalize appropriate removal of electrode. To detach the electrode, rotate the electrode counter-clockwise until it is free from the fetal presenting part. Do not pull the electrode from the fetal skin. Document electrode removed intact.

Spiral Electrode

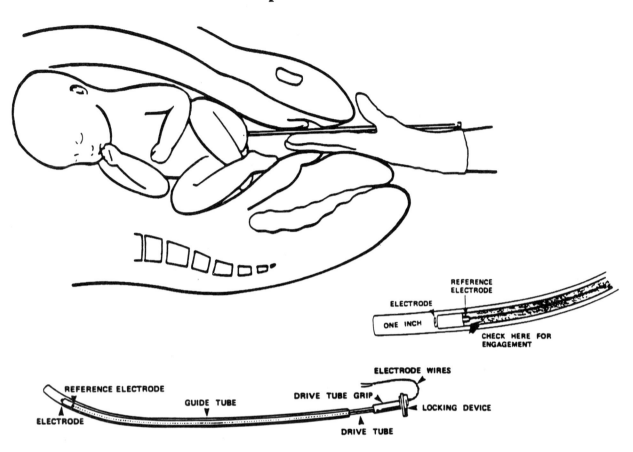

Electrode placement -- breech presentation

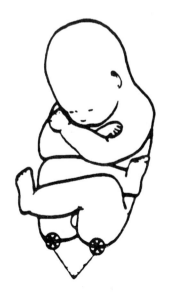

Electrode placement sites -- sites presentation

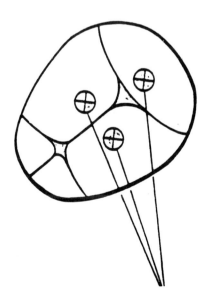

Electrode placement -- cephalic

2. <u>Intrauterine Pressure Catheter Placement</u>:

This is a direct method of measuring the uterine activity during labor and the <u>only</u> method of measuring uterine <u>intensity</u> or <u>strength</u>. It is measured in millimeters of mercury, mm Hg, and is useful at any altitude.

<u>Procedure</u>:

(1) Prepare IUPC per type and instruction of the manufacturer.

(2) Set up IUPC. (Verbalizes sterile technique and donning gloves.)

    (a)   Assemble equipment, attach IUPC to adaptor cable.

    (b)   Verbalize flushing transducer and catheter, if fluid-filled.

    (c)   Verbalize flushing of IUPC syringe, if fluid-filled.

    (d)   Verbalize zeroing monitor while open to air.

(3) Determine cervical site for catheter insertion, gently displace presenting part, if needed.

(4) Insert guide (containing IUPC) between examining fingers.

(5) Ensure catheter guide does not extend beyond fingers.

(6) Insert until 45 cm or until resistance is met (do not force IUPC).

(7) Verbalize attaching to cable and assuring proper functioning.

(8) Verbalize that documentation on tracing and medical record is completed.

Intrauterine Pressure Catheter

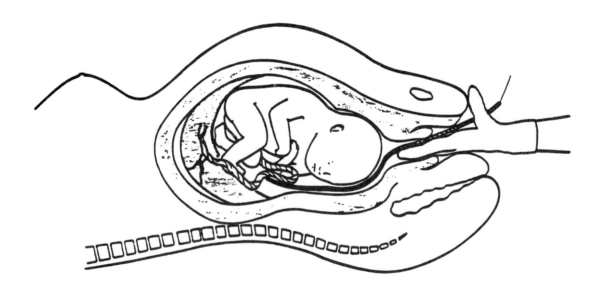

Critical Errors in Testing:

1. Failure to simulate all steps in procedures.

2. Failure to demonstrate safety principles related to placement.

3. Failure to demonstrate correct sequence of steps in placement.

Evaluation:

SKILL EVALUATION: **Instrumentation**

A. Fetal Spiral Electrode Placement

	Pass	**Fail**	**Date**
1. Verbalizes procedure to mother prior to application.	_____	_____	_____
2. Verbalizes opening electrode package and donning gloves.	_____	_____	_____
3. Removes wires from between drive tube and guide tube.	_____	_____	_____
4. Pulls electrode one inch back into guide tube so it does not extend beyond end of guide.	_____	_____	_____
5. Performs vaginal exam, assesses presenting part, feels for firm bone and avoids face, fontanel, genitalia; maintains fingers on target areas.	_____	_____	_____
6. Places guide tube between two examining fingers and firmly places against fetal head at a right angle.	_____	_____	_____
7. Advances drive tube until it touches the presenting part.	_____	_____	_____
8. Maintains pressure against presenting part and turns clockwise (about 1 ½ times) until resistance is met.	_____	_____	_____
9. Releases lock device and slides guides of electrode.	_____	_____	_____
10. Checks placement of electrode before withdrawing examining fingers.	_____	_____	_____
11. Verbalizes attaching monitor to cable device.	_____	_____	_____
12. Verbalizes that cable is plugged into monitor.	_____	_____	_____
13. Verbalizes appropriate removal of electrode.	_____	_____	_____

B. Intrauterine Pressure Catheter Placement

	Pass	Fail	Date
1. Prepares IUPC per type and instruction of the manufacturer.	_____	_____	_____
2. Sets up IUPC.			
a. Assembles equipment, attaches to adaptor cable	_____	_____	_____
b. Verbalizes flushing transducer, if fluid-filled	_____	_____	_____
c. Verbalizes flushing IUPC syringe, if fluid-filled	_____	_____	_____
d. Verbalizes zeroing monitor while open to air	_____	_____	_____
3. Determines cervical site for catheter insertion, gently displacing presenting part, if needed.	_____	_____	_____
4. Inserts guide (containing IUPC) between examining fingers. (Note: Some models may not use a guide.)	_____	_____	_____
5. Ensures catheter guide does not extend beyond fingers.	_____	_____	_____
6. Inserts until 45 cm or until resistance is met (does not force IUPC).	_____	_____	_____
7. Verbalizes attaching to cable and assuring proper functioning.	_____	_____	_____
8. Verbalizes that documentation on tracing and medical record is completed.	_____	_____	_____

Special thanks is extended to Utah Medical for sponsoring the revisions to the "Spiral Electrode and Intrauterine Pressure Catheter Placement" video. Thanks also goes to Graphic Controls for their donation of fetal monitoring spiral electrodes and to Utah Medical for their donation of intrauterine pressure catheters.

Integration of Fetal Heart Monitoring Knowledge and Skills

Objectives:

In this skill station, the participant will

1. Demonstrate appropriate interpretation of the fetal monitor tracing.

2. Describe the physiologic mechanisms for the observed patterns.

3. State instrumentation factors affecting interpretation of the fetal monitor tracing.

4. Integrate physiologic rationales and interpretation into the decision-making process.

5. Specify appropriate interventions or management steps for each case scenario.

6. Evaluate fetal response to selected interventions.

Introductory Principles:

1. A systematic review of the fetal monitor tracings provides the basis for determining appropriate responses or interventions to be initiated.

2. The fetal monitor tracing should be interpreted in light of the maternal/fetal historical and physical assessment data.

3. The physiology of pregnancy and labor is a dynamic process. Integration of physiologic-based data must account for changes from previous physiologic states. Decision-making and interventions should project for future physiologic changes. Each maternal/fetal unit presents along a physiologic continuum, which forms the basis for the logical progression from interpretation to integration to decision-making to evaluation.

4. Physiologic goals and supportive actions:

Improve uterine blood flow
- maternal position change
- hydration
- medication
- anxiety reduction

Improve oxygenation
- maternal position change
- maternal oxygen
- maternal breathing techniques

Improve umbilical circulation
- maternal position change
- vaginal manipulation
- amnioinfusion

Reduce uterine activity
- maternal position change
- hydration
- modified pushing
- medication

5. Although there is not always universal agreement on whether specific patterns are reassuring or nonreassuring, there is a clear understanding that based on the interpretation of certain fetal responses (e.g., variable decelerations, variability changes), actions are indicated. Remember to respond to the likely physiologic etiology.

6. Additional actions to be considered include further assessments (e.g., scalp stimulation), troubleshooting of equipment, notification of care providers, and documentation.

7. Monitoring methods have improved over the years. However, external and internal modes of monitoring do have certain limitations which may affect interpretation.

8. Evaluation includes reassessing to determine whether there is a need to continue, alter, or discontinue interventions based on observed responses.

Steps in Skill Performance:

Consider that integration of all information is the purpose of this exercise, including history, findings, physiology, monitoring modes, interpretation, interventions, and evaluation. Each participant will be given time to review and discuss patient histories and practice tracings. Verbal responses are appropriate for practice sessions, while written responses to the fetal monitor tracings will be expected during testing.

1. Review pertinent patient history.

2. Interpret the monitor tracing for fetal heart baseline rate, variability, periodic and nonperiodic changes.

3. Interpret the uterine activity patterns.

4. Describe possible physiologic mechanisms for patterns (e.g., adequate oxygen reserves; inadequate uterine, placental, or cord blood flow; fetal response to nervous system stimulation or movement or cord compression).

5. State instrumentation factors which may affect interpretation of the tracings.

6. List intervention and management steps based on integration of history, interpretation of data, and physiologic responses.

7. Evaluate fetal response to interventions.

Critical Errors in Testing:

1. Failure to correctly interpret FHR, variability and appropriate characteristics (e.g., periodic and nonperiodic patterns).

2. Failure to correctly interpret uterine activity characteristics.

3. Failure to identify physiologic factors which could contribute to the observed patterns.

4. Failure to recognize limitations of the monitoring method.

5. Failure to consider pertinent history.

6. Failure to select intended physiologic goal(s) and critical interventions based on interpretation.

Evaluation:

SKILL EVALUATION: **Integration of Fetal Heart Monitoring Knowledge and Skills**

	Pass	**Fail**	**Date**
1. Interprets the components of the FHR tracing (FHR baseline, long-term and short-term variability as appropriate, periodic changes by name when present, nonperiodic changes by name when present).	_____	_____	_____
2. Interprets uterine contraction patterns based on monitoring mode (frequency, duration, intensity, resting tone).	_____	_____	_____
3. States underlying physiologic mechanisms for observed patterns.	_____	_____	_____
4. Lists three critical management steps or interventions for each tracing segment (including troubleshooting instrumentation).	_____	_____	_____
5. Evaluates fetal responses to interventions.	_____	_____	_____

Communication of Fetal Heart Monitoring Data

Objectives:

In this skill station, the participant will

1. Critique a videotaped scenario of nurse-physician communication. List four omissions in the nurse-physician video.

2. Document an accurate interpretation of a selected fetal monitor tracing. Correctly document baseline rate, FHR variability (LTV and STV, if appropriate), periodic and nonperiodic fetal heart patterns, and uterine activity on the flowsheet. Document on long notes, if appropriate.

3. Document the plan of action for responding to a situation of conflict.

4. Reproduce a fetal monitor tracing from written documentation using blank fetal monitor paper.

Introductory Principles:

Communication is the process by which we understand others and endeavor to be understood by them. It is dynamic, constantly changing, and shifting in response to the total situation.

The nurse caring for a maternity patient must possess excellent communication skills. Whether communication is verbal, nonverbal, or recorded, it must be accurate, objective, and concise.

Briefly review expectations for each type of communication. Practice the below steps as needed. The video exercise will be tested first following the group viewing. The remainder will be tested at your own pace so that all three exercises will be completed within the time allotted.

Steps in Skill Performance:

Steps of Communication with the Physician

1. Clarify the identity of the nurse initiating the communication as well as where the communication is originating (name of hospital) and then the identity of the patient being discussed.

2. Clarify the purpose of the conversation or call (e.g., to report an update of progress, obtain an order, ask questions, state concerns, or request physician presence).

3. Provide a clear, concise review of the patient's history and her status. More detail is needed if physician is covering for someone else or does not know the patient very well. If requested to do actions which are against hospital policy, advise that it is not possible to do so and offer an alternative when possible. For example, " I cannot give IV medication without an access to the vein, but I can give it through a heparin lock or infusion," or "I cannot rupture membranes, but Dr. _____ is here. Would you like to talk with Dr. _____?"

If requested to perform an action which seems inappropriate for the situation, state your discomfort and reason. If a conflict remains, tell the physician you will notify your supervisor first.

4. Write a telephone order in clear terms and repeat back to the physician when possible. Date and time the order and ensure its legibility as well as its compliance with hospital protocol, e.g. "T.O. _____/_____."

5. Document the time of the conversation with the physician and the purpose or outcome in the patient record. For example, "Dr. _____ notified of patient's vaginal exam and EFM pattern." In this case, the patient's record will contain documentation of the EFM pattern and vaginal examination which will coincide with that reported to the physician. "Dr. _____ requested to come for delivery." The notes contain only action information, not details about the conversation. Each hospital has a protocol for recording the actual conversation when necessary such as a QAR form or incident report. The nurse should be familiar with these protocols and forms.

Steps of Communication with the Patient

1. Explain events and procedures to the patient in understandable terms (at the level of the patient's understanding), without extreme detail or brevity.

2. Ask whether the patient has any questions.

3. Answer questions and refer to the physician, certified nurse midwife, or other appropriate person when necessary.

4. Listen to concerns, fears, requests, and other questions from the patient and her support person(s).

5. Respond with answers, reassurance, and explanations. Refer to the physician, certified nurse-midwife, or others when necessary.

6. Document patient teaching, patient responses, and patient problems.

Steps of Communication with Another Nurse

1. Identify patient(s) discussed clearly.

2. Convey urgent and stat requests or information directly, clearly, and as calmly as possible.

3. Provide complete, clear patient care information and other information, such as the physician's or certified nurse-midwife's location and the support person's presence and demeanor.

4. Convey strategies that were particularly successful or unsuccessful for patient care continuity.

<u>Guidelines in Recording FHM Information</u>

1. When charting auscultated or palpated information, include the audible rate and rhythm as well as whether decreases or increases were present.

2. Documentation of EFM data includes the baseline range (unless uninterpretable), accelerations and decelerations, and uterine activity according to the capability of the equipment. For example, the spiral electrode will provide different data than the ultrasound.

3. The documentation reflects the trend of the pattern as opposed to recording each deceleration or acceleration.

4. The documentation also describes the events so that they could be reasonably understood if the tracing is mislabeled or lost (hard copy or disk) or incomplete.

5. Document the components of a pattern, such as the type of deceleration. If there is controversy regarding a deceleration pattern, a description may be helpful. If a description of the pattern is documented, include shape, the range of the deceleration depth (nadir), duration of the nadir, recovery time from the end of the nadir to the baseline (or other rate), and baseline variability (LTV and STV).

Critical Errors in Testing:

1. Failure to document accurately an interpretation of the tracing including

    *   Baseline FHR
    *   FHR variability (LTV and STV, if appropriate)
    *   Appropriate FHR characteristics (e.g., nonperiodic and periodic patterns)
    *   Uterine activity.

2. Failure to document appropriate plan of action when physician's or midwife's order causes conflict.

3. Failure to list four omissions in the video of nurse-physician reporting.

4. Failure to validate omissions critical to the final outcome.

5. Failure to reproduce uterine and fetal tracing from written nursing documentation on the blank fetal monitor paper provided.*

---

*   Note: The intention of reproducing a tracing is to highlight the importance of clarity of documentation.

Evaluation:

SKILL EVALUATION: **Communication of Fetal Heart Monitoring Data**

		Pass	**Fail**	**Date**
1.	Critiques videotaped communication noting four omissions.	_____	_____	_____
2.	Documents accurate interpretation of selected fetal monitor tracing.	_____	_____	_____
3.	Documents appropriate plan of action in response to situation of conflict.	_____	_____	_____
4.	Reproduces uterine and fetal tracing from written nursing documentation.	_____	_____	_____

Special thanks is extended to Donna Adelsperger, RNC, MEd, and the staff at Bethesda Hospitals, Inc., Cincinnati, OH, for their help in developing materials used in this skill station.

CHAPTER 10: CASE STUDY EXERCISES

Introduction

The FHMPP workshop uses the analysis of case studies to examine the nursing approach to fetal heart monitoring in the care of intrapartum patients. Two case study exercises are included to provide an orientation to the method of interpretation of fetal heart and uterine activity tracings, identification of the physiologic significance of the pattern observed, and decision-making for interventions used in the workshop. Review of these case studies prior to the workshop is recommended.

For each case exercise, review the segment of tracing and brief history provided and complete the case data form. Correctly completed case data forms are provided beginning on page 258. In the clinical setting and in the course skill station, longer segments of tracing are used for interpretation and decision making for interventions.

AWHONN FETAL HEART MONITORING PRINCIPLES AND PRACTICES
SYSTEMATIC APPROACH TO INTERPRETATION WORKSHEET

Case Study Exercise #_____

1. Contractions: Frequency   _____
                       Duration   _____
                       Intensity   _____
                       Resting tonus   _____

2. Baseline FHR: _____

3. Variability: Place a check signifying the appropriate type of variability on the strip.

                    LTV   a.   decreased (0-5 bpm)   _____
                           b.   average (6-25 bpm)   _____
                           c.   marked (>25 bpm)   _____
                           d.   unable to assess   _____

                    STV   a.   present   _____
                           b.   absent   _____
                           c.   unable to assess   _____

4. Accelerations and decelerations: When present, circle P if _periodic_ and NP if _nonperiodic_.

    Accelerations   P   NP
    Early decelerations   P
    Variable decelerations   P   NP
    Late decelerations   P
    Prolonged decelerations   P   NP

5. List possible underlying physiologic mechanism/rationales for observed pattern.

6. List the most immediate physiologic goal(s) you are trying to achieve based on the observed pattern.

7. List actions to achieve the physiologic goals, and list actions needed related to instrumentation or further assessment.

Case Study Exercise #1

Patient History

Fiona is a 32 year old woman, gravida 4, para 2012, who is at 39 weeks of gestation. Her family and personal medical history show no risk factors. She experienced one miscarriage. She has two living children and experienced no complications with those pregnancies. With this pregnancy, she has developed pregnancy-induced hypertension. Her nonstress test yesterday was reactive but several variable decelerations, not associated with uterine contractions, were noted. Her biophysical profile score was 8/10 with decreased amniotic fluid volume (and the reactive nonstress test). She was admitted to Labor and Delivery for Pitocin induction of labor at 7:00 a.m. today. She is 2-3 cm dilated, 50% effaced, and at a -2 station on admission. Her vital signs are as follows: blood pressure 132/94 (pre-pregnant blood pressure 110/78), pulse 80, respiration 20, and temperature 97.8° F (36.5° C). Laboratory values are within normal limits. At 10:40 a.m., she is 5 cm dilated, 80% effaced, and at a -2 station. Spontaneous rupture of membranes occurs at 11:25 a.m. with meconium stained fluid. A spiral electrode was inserted. Upon vaginal exam, she is 6 cm dilated and at -1 station. Her blood pressure is 136/94 and her pulse is 90.

Case Study Exercise #1

Tracing Segment A

This tracing takes place at 11:40 a.m. Monitor mode: Spiral electrode/Toco

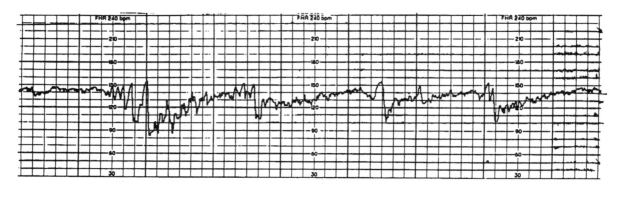

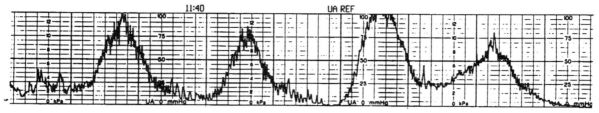

AWHONN FETAL HEART MONITORING PRINCIPLES AND PRACTICES
SYSTEMATIC APPROACH TO INTERPRETATION WORKSHEET

Case Study Exercise # 1, segment A

1. Contractions: Frequency   _____
                      Duration   _____
                      Intensity   _____
                      Resting tonus _____

2. Baseline FHR: _____

3. Variability: Place a check signifying the appropriate type of variability on the strip.

                LTV   a. decreased (0-5 bpm)   _____
                       b. average (6-25 bpm)   _____
                       c. marked (>25 bpm)   _____
                       d. unable to assess   _____

                STV   a. present   _____
                       b. absent   _____
                       c. unable to assess   _____

4. Accelerations and decelerations: When present, circle P if periodic and NP if nonperiodic.

    Accelerations   P   NP
    Early decelerations   P
    Variable decelerations   P   NP
    Late decelerations   P
    Prolonged decelerations   P   NP

5. List possible underlying physiologic mechanism/rationales for observed pattern.

6. List the most immediate physiologic goal(s) you are trying to achieve based on the observed pattern.

7. List actions to achieve the physiologic goals, and list actions needed related to instrumentation or further assessment.

Case Study Exercise #1

Tracing Segment B

This tracing takes place at 11:50 a.m. Monitor mode: Spiral electrode/Toco

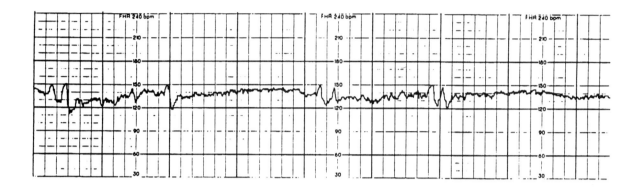

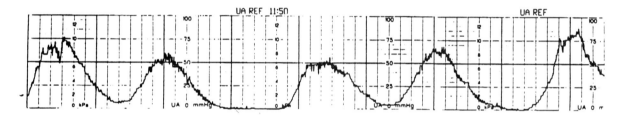

AWHONN FETAL HEART MONITORING PRINCIPLES AND PRACTICES
SYSTEMATIC APPROACH TO INTERPRETATION WORKSHEET

Case Study Exercise # <u>1, segment B</u>

1. Contractions: Frequency   _____
                      Duration   _____
                      Intensity   _____
                      Resting tonus   _____

2. Baseline FHR: _____

3. Variability: Place a check signifying the appropriate type of variability on the strip.

                  LTV   a.   decreased (0-5 bpm)   _____
                         b.   average (6-25 bpm)   _____
                         c.   marked (>25 bpm)   _____
                         d.   unable to assess   _____

                  STV   a.   present   _____
                         b.   absent   _____
                         c.   unable to assess   _____

4. Accelerations and decelerations: When present, circle P if <u>periodic</u> and NP if <u>nonperiodic</u>.

    Accelerations   P   NP
    Early decelerations   P
    Variable decelerations   P   NP
    Late decelerations   P
    Prolonged decelerations   P   NP

5. List possible underlying physiologic mechanism/rationales for observed pattern.

6. List the most immediate physiologic goal(s) you are trying to achieve based on the observed pattern.

7. List actions to achieve the physiologic goals, and list actions needed related to instrumentation or further assessment.

251

Case Study Exercise #1

Tracing Segment C
This tracing takes place at 12 noon. Monitor mode: Spiral electrode/Toco

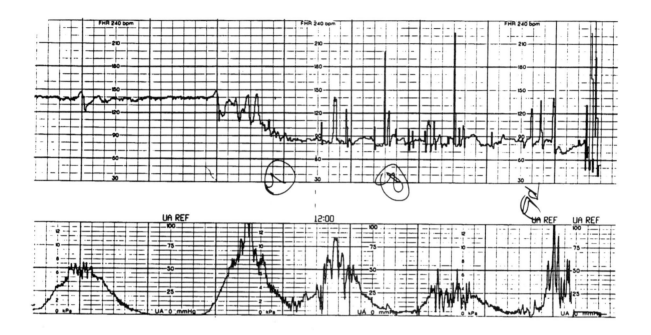

AWHONN FETAL HEART MONITORING PRINCIPLES AND PRACTICES
SYSTEMATIC APPROACH TO INTERPRETATION WORKSHEET

Case Study Exercise # <u>1, segment C</u>

1. Contractions: Frequency   _____
                      Duration   _____
                      Intensity   _____
                      Resting tonus   _____

2. Baseline FHR: _____

3. Variability: Place a check signifying the appropriate type of variability on the strip.

                  LTV   a.   decreased (0-5 bpm)   _____
                         b.   average (6-25 bpm)   _____
                         c.   marked (>25 bpm)   _____
                         d.   unable to assess   _____

                  STV   a.   present   _____
                         b.   absent   _____
                         c.   unable to assess   _____

4. Accelerations and decelerations: When present, circle P if <u>periodic</u> and NP if <u>nonperiodic</u>.

    Accelerations   P   NP
    Early decelerations   P
    Variable decelerations   P   NP
    Late decelerations   P
    Prolonged decelerations   P   NP

5. List possible underlying physiologic mechanism/rationales for observed pattern.

6. List the most immediate physiologic goal(s) you are trying to achieve based on the observed pattern.

7. List actions to achieve the physiologic goals, and list actions needed related to instrumentation or further assessment.

Case Study Exercise #2

Patient History

Abigail is a 20 year old woman, gravida 1, para 0, at 40 $^2/_7$ weeks of gestation. Her past medical and family history shows no risk factors. During this pregnancy her blood pressure has ranged from 110/70 to 130/84. Sonograms were done three times, and results were consistent with dates and fundal heights. She has been admitted to Labor and Delivery stating her contractions are "uncomfortable." A vaginal exam reveals the cervix is 1-2 cm dilated and 90% effaced, with a vertex at 0 station, and intact membranes. Artificial rupture of membranes with thick meconium noted was done shortly after admission.

Case Study Exercise #2

This tracing takes place at 1 hour after admission. Monitor mode: Ultrasound/Toco

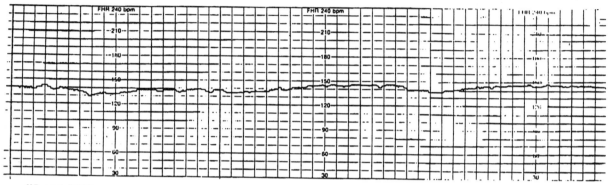

US and TOCO

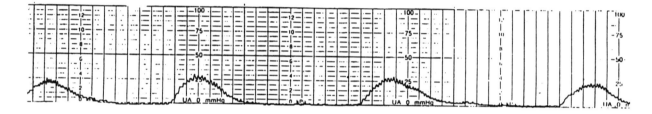

AWHONN FETAL HEART MONITORING PRINCIPLES AND PRACTICES
SYSTEMATIC APPROACH TO INTERPRETATION WORKSHEET

Case Study Exercise # <u>2</u>

1.   Contractions: Frequency   _____
                      Duration   _____
                      Intensity   _____
                      Resting tonus   _____

2.   Baseline FHR: _____

3.   Variability: Place a check signifying the appropriate type of variability on the strip.

                 LTV   a.   decreased (0-5 bpm)   _____
                        b.   average (6-25 bpm)   _____
                        c.   marked (>25 bpm)   _____
                        d.   unable to assess   _____

                 STV   a.   present   _____
                        b.   absent   _____
                        c.   unable to assess   _____

4.   Accelerations and decelerations: When present, circle P if <u>periodic</u> and NP if <u>nonperiodic</u>.

     Accelerations   P   NP
     Early decelerations   P
     Variable decelerations   P   NP
     Late decelerations   P
     Prolonged decelerations   P   NP

5.   List possible underlying physiologic mechanism/rationales for observed pattern.

6.   List the most immediate physiologic goal(s) you are trying to achieve based on the observed pattern.

7.   List actions to achieve the physiologic goals, and list actions needed related to instrumentation or further assessment.

257

Answers to Case Study Exercises

AWHONN FETAL HEART MONITORING PRINCIPLES AND PRACTICES

Systematic Approach to Interpretation Worksheet

Case Study Exercise # 1, segment A

1. Contractions: Frequency   q 1½-2 min
                      Duration   75-80 seconds with coupling
                      Intensity   palpation
                      Resting tonus   palpation

2. Baseline FHR: 130-150 bpm

3. Variability: LTV   a.   decreased (0-5 bpm)   _____
                           b.   average (6-25 bpm)   ____✔_____
                           c.   marked (>25 bpm)   _____
                           d.   unable to assess   _____

                    STV   a.   present   ____✔_____
                           b.   absent   _____
                           c.   unable to assess   _____

4. Accelerations and decelerations: When present, circle P if periodic and NP if nonperiodic.

Accelerations	P	NP
Early decelerations	P	
Variable decelerations	ⓟ	NP
Late decelerations	P	
Prolonged decelerations	P	NP

5. List possible underlying physiologic mechanism/rationales for observed pattern.

    • Contractions may be hypertonic and increased in frequency and resting tonus related to oxytocin induction.

    • Variable decelerations related to umbilical cord compression (baroreceptor and parasympathetic responses); decreased amniotic fluid volume may be a factor in cord compression with resultant decreased cushioning effect; if patient is progressing, may also be associated with descent of fetus (second stage variable decelerations).

    • The fetus is demonstrating reserves as evidenced by the presence of STV and LTV after recovery from the variable decelerations. Brief acceleratory responses (shoulders) in the FHR also present prior to decelerations.

6. List the most immediate physiologic goal(s) you are trying to achieve based on the observed pattern.

    - Reduce uterine activity
    - Improve umbilical circulation

7. List actions to achieve the physiologic goals, and list actions needed related to instrumentation or further assessment.

    - Promote umbilical circulation through maternal position change and perform vaginal exam, as indicated, to check for presence of prolapsed cord.
    - Reduce uterine activity; decrease Pitocin, position patient laterally.
    - Adjust tocodynamometer, as necessary.
    - If pattern worsens, may consider amnioinfusion (depending on total clinical picture, progress in labor, and institutional policy).
    - Observe for tocodynamometer response to interventions.

AWHONN FETAL HEART MONITORING PRINCIPLES AND PRACTICES

Systematic Approach to Interpretation Worksheet

Case Study Exercise # 1, segment B

1. Contractions: Frequency   1½-2 minutes
                       Duration   75-80 seconds
                       Intensity   palpation
                       Resting tonus   palpation

2. Baseline FHR: 130-145 bpm

3. Variability: LTV   a.   decreased (0-5 bpm)   _____
                           b.   average (6-25 bpm)   ____✔_____
                           c.   marked (>25 bpm)   _____
                           d.   unable to assess   _____

                    STV   a.   present   ____✔_____
                           b.   absent   _____
                           c.   unable to assess   _____

4. Accelerations and decelerations: When present, circle P if periodic and NP if nonperiodic.

    Accelerations   P   NP
    Early decelerations   P
    Variable decelerations   ⓟ   NP
    Late decelerations   P
    Prolonged decelerations   P   NP

5. List possible underlying physiologic mechanism/rationales for observed pattern.

    •   Position change has decreased the variable decelerations. May still be partial compression of
               the umbilical vein with resultant accelerations ("shoulders") associated with possible chemore-
               ceptor and sympathetic nervous system response.
    •   Fetus continues to demonstrate reserves (STV).
    •   Coupling of contractions with oxytocin.

6. List the most immediate physiologic goal(s) you are trying to achieve based on the observed pattern.

    •   Reduce uterine activity

7. List actions to achieve the physiologic goals, and list actions needed related to instrumentation or further assessment.

- Decrease oxytocin, palpate uterus.
- Continue to assess fetal heart response.
- Continue routine assessments and interventions for labor.

AWHONN FETAL HEART MONITORING PRINCIPLES AND PRACTICES

Systematic Approach to Interpretation Worksheet

Case Study Exercise # <u>1, segment C</u>

1. Contractions: Frequency   <u>q 1½-2½ minutes</u>
                    Duration   <u>70-80 seconds</u>
                    Intensity   <u>palpation</u>
                    Resting tonus <u>palpation</u>

2. Baseline FHR: <u>135-140 bpm, then 75-90 bpm</u>

3. Variability: LTV a. decreased (0-5 bpm)   _____✔_____ (When FHR is 135-140)
                       b. average (6-25 bpm)   _____✔_____ (When FHR is 75-90)
                       c. marked (>25 bpm)   _____
                       d. unable to assess   _____

                  STV a. present   _____✔_____
                       b. absent   _____
                       c. unable to assess   _____

4. Accelerations and decelerations: When present, circle P if <u>periodic</u> and NP if <u>nonperiodic</u>.

    Accelerations   P   NP
    Early decelerations   P
    Variable decelerations Ⓟ   NP
    Late decelerations   P
    Prolonged decelerations P   ⓃⓅ

5. List possible underlying physiologic mechanism/rationales for observed pattern.

    •   Umbilical cord compression, possible rapid fetal descent and impending delivery, stretching or
            tightening of the umbilical cord with head compression and vagal response, possible prolapse
            of cord with related baroreceptor and vagal response.
    •   Prolonged deceleration also may be related to increased uterine activity and decreased resting
            period.

262

6. List the most immediate physiologic goal(s) you are trying to achieve based on the observed pattern.

    - Improve umbilical circulation
    - Reduce uterine activity
    - Improve oxygenation
    - Improve uterine blood flow

7. List actions to achieve the physiologic goals, and list actions needed related to instrumentation or further assessment.

    - Improve umbilical and uterine blood flow with maternal position change(s). Hydrate with IV plasma expander.
    - Decrease uterine activity by turning Pitocin off (and repositioning laterally).
    - Oxygenate with maternal oxygen via tight mask.
    - Quickly assess for possible causes while intervening (e.g., vaginal exam to rule out umbilical cord prolapse or to elevate presenting part if cord present; vital signs to rule out hypotension).
    - Notify primary care provider and neonatal team.
    - Prepare for possible delivery.
    - Observe fetal response to scalp stimulation on vaginal examination after recovery of FHR.
    - Continue further actions and assessments if FHR remains bradycardic.

OUTCOME:

No cord was felt on vaginal examination. The patient dilated rapidly and a normal spontaneous vaginal delivery took place 8 minutes later. Apgar scores were 8 and 9. The umbilical artery pH was 7.28, reflective of a non-acidotic fetus with reserves demonstrated by prior presence of accelerations and variability.

AWHONN FETAL HEART MONITORING PRINCIPLES AND PRACTICES

Systematic Approach to Interpretation Worksheet

Case Study Exercise # 2

1. Contractions:

Frequency	q 2-3 minutes
Duration	60-70 seconds
Intensity	palpation
Resting tonus	palpation

2. Baseline FHR: 140-145 bpm

3. Variability:

LTV
a. decreased (0-5 bpm) ✔
b. average (6-25 bpm) _____
c. marked (>25 bpm) _____
d. unable to assess _____

STV
a. present _____
b. absent _____
c. unable to assess ✔ *unable to rely on ultrasound;
however, likely to be absent with spiral electrode.

4. Accelerations and decelerations: When present, circle P if periodic and NP if nonperiodic.

Accelerations	P	NP
Early decelerations	P	
Variable decelerations	P	NP
Late decelerations	Ⓟ	
Prolonged decelerations	P	NP

5. List possible underlying physiologic mechanism/rationales for observed pattern.

• Late decelerations related to uteroplacental insufficiency. May be related to placental factors (such as aging of placenta, infarcts, calcification, small surface area), maternal factors (such as maternal hypotension, supine positioning, medication, decreased maternal oxygenation), or fetal factors (such as possible anemia). Although sonograms have indicated normal fetal growth, possible placental changes may have occurred associated with elevations in maternal blood pressure (PIH).

• Presence of thick meconium may be associated with hypoxic insult.

• Decreased variability (LTV and likely absent STV, in particular) may indicate loss of fetal reserves, increasing the likelihood that these are not reflex late decelerations.

264

6. List the most immediate physiologic goal(s) you are trying to achieve based on the observed pattern.

   - Reduce uterine activity
   - Improve oxygenation
   - Improve uterine blood flow

7. List actions to achieve the physiologic goals, and list actions needed related to instrumentation or further assessment.

   - Reposition laterally to increase maternal cardiac output and uterine blood flow.
   - Provide oxygen via tight face mask to increase maternal/fetal oxygenation.
   - Hydrate, as indicated, with plasma expander to increase maternal blood volume and increase uteroplacental blood flow.
   - Decrease uterine activity (e.g., turn off Pitocin, if on; reposition laterally; consider tocolytic, as indicated). Palpate contractions.
   - Notify primary care provider, neonatal team, and anesthesiologist.
   - Vaginal examination to determine progress (was only 1 cm dilated).
   - Prepare for alternate route of delivery.
   - Provide support to decrease maternal anxiety and catecholamine response.
   - Observe for bleeding or signs of abruption.
   - Observe fetal heart rate responses to interventions.

OUTCOME:

A cesarean section was performed one-half hour later. Apgar scores were 3 and 8 with intubation at birth to evaluate whether meconium was below the vocal cords. Umbilical artery pH of 7.15 and decreased PO_2 indicated the presence of metabolic acidosis.

INDEX OF FIGURES AND TABLES

INDEX OF KEY TERMS